Chronic Obstructive
Pulmonary Disease
in Primary Care

Chronic Obstructive Pulmonary Disease in Primary Care

All you need to know to manage COPD in your practice

Dr David Bellamy MBE, BSc, FRCP, MRCGP, DRCOG

GP Principal with a special interest in respiratory medicine at the James Fisher Medical Centre, Bournemouth Member of the COPD Guidelines Committee

and

Rachel Booker RGN DN(Cert)HV

COPD course leader for the National Asthma and Respiratory Training Centre, Warwick

Class Health • London

Printing history
First published 2000
Reprinted 2000

The authors and publishers welcome feedback from the users of this book.
Please contact the publishers:

Class Publishing (London) Ltd,
Barb House, Barb Mews,
London W6 7PA
Telephone: (020) 7371 2119;
Fax (020) 7371 2878 [International +4420]

A CIP catalogue record for this book is available from the British Library

ISBN 1-872362-95-8

Edited by Gillian Clarke

Index by Valerie Elliston

Produced by Landmark Production Consultants Ltd, Princes Risborough

Designed and typeset by Martin Bristow

Printed and bound in Slovenia by printing house Delo Tiskarna
by arrangement with Korotan Ljubljana

Contents

Acknowledgements

We thank Greta Barnes, Director of the National Asthma and Respiratory Training Centre, and Richard Harrison, consultant respiratory physician at Stockton on Tees. Without their encouragement, this book would never have been started.

We also thank Glynis Bellamy, for her help with word processing parts of the manuscript, and to both our families for their support and tolerance.

Foreword
by Greta Barnes, MBE
Director of the National Asthma and Respiratory Training Centre

In recent years alterations in health care and health policy have accelerated change in the management of chronic diseases such as diabetes, asthma and hypertension. There has been an increasing shift of emphasis from secondary to primary care, and a collaborative approach has been encouraged not only between hospital and general practice but also between GP and practice nurse.

By 2020 chronic obstructive pulmonary disease (COPD), the 'smokers' disease', is likely to become the UK's fifth most common cause of death. It will also be managed chiefly in the community. At present it has been acknowledged that COPD is not widely understood by the vast majority of doctors and nurses, particularly in primary care. Many patients may have been misdiagnosed and therefore inappropriately treated.

The publication of *Chronic Obstructive Pulmonary Disease in Primary Care* is very timely. It provides a wealth of practical information for all health professionals who work in general practice. The authors highlight the importance of correct diagnosis and the value of spirometry as well as how to treat and manage the patient with COPD. The chapter on smoking cessation, which is the single most important intervention, provides invaluable advice to the reader, as does the section on ways to improve the quality of life for patients with this debilitating condition.

David Bellamy and Rachel Booker have a wealth of experience looking after COPD patients in general practice. In this book they have demonstrated the value of combining medical and nursing experience so that they can help others strive for excellence.

Undoubtedly this book will attract a wide range of health professionals who work in the community. It will also serve admirably to complement the National Asthma and Respiratory Training Centre's Chronic Obstructive Pulmonary Disease Training Programme.

The authors are to be congratulated on producing a much-needed book – the first of its kind for primary care.

Foreword

by Professor Peter Calverley, MB, FRCP, FRCPE
Professor of Medicine (Pulmonary and Rehabilitation),
The University of Liverpool

Chronic obstructive pulmonary disease is a common, often unrecognised, source of morbidity and mortality in the UK and throughout
the world. Traditionally, it has been seen as a 'dull' condition devoid
of exciting symptoms or physical signs that help enliven the teaching
of medical students and largely unresponsive to treatment. This
therapeutic failure on the doctor's part is often excused by the
recognition that the condition itself is usually brought on by cigarette smoking and therefore is 'the patient's own fault'. This has led
to a type of therapeutic nihilism, which can no longer be justified
given the changes in our understanding of the causes and consequences of COPD as well as the availability of more effective
treatments. Despite encouraging reductions in the use of cigarettes,
especially by middle-aged men, the problems of the COPD patient
persist and are likely to do so even in the developed economies of
the world. Patients who might have succumbed from their illness
had they continued smoking in the past now develop symptoms
related to their previous lung damage as they age, and this respiratory disability is an increasing burden to all those involved in the
care of older patients. We now have the techniques relatively readily
available to help make a firm diagnosis of COPD and to distinguish
these patients from the many others with a bewildering array of
similar symptoms produced by different pathologies, where the
therapeutic approach and the likely prognosis will vary. The management of the COPD patient is increasingly multidisciplinary and
the patients themselves are entitled to explanations not only of how
their disease arises but also what the different treatments recommended do and what kind of improvement they are likely to
achieve. The dilemma for health professionals is that this type of
information has often not been available to them during their training, nor is it sufficiently up to date to help them form a useful
management plan. This book has set out to remedy these problems.

This short book provides a wealth of information and practical
advice, based on clinical experience and evidence-based recommendations. It is written by a general practitioner and a nurse educator,
both with wide experience of respiratory disease and who are famil-
iar with the kinds of questions that someone new to this field is

bound to ask. They stress the importance of a positive diagnosis and of a positive therapeutic approach. When the correct patients are identified, useful things can be done for them even if this is unlikely to completely abolish all their symptoms once the disease itself is advanced.

The authors have been keen to demystify the role of pulmonary function testing while indicating how it fits into everyday clinical management. Their recommendations are up to date, and include some of the very latest clinical trial data as well as practical comments about the management of complications and acute exacerbations of disease. The result is a handbook of practical information that will be helpful to everyone concerned with this common clinical problem.

Hopefully, those who read and use this book will feel more confident about managing COPD in their daily practice, which in turn will begin to reverse the expectations of patients and doctors that, in the past, have been so low but no longer need to be quite so pessimistic.

Abbreviations

AHR airway hyper-responsiveness

AMP adenosine monophosphate

BMI body mass index

BTS British Thoracic Society

CT computed tomography

FEV$_1$ forced expired volume produced in the first second

FEV$_1$/FVC% the ratio of FEV$_1$ to FVC, expressed as a percentage

FVC forced vital capacity – the total volume of air that can be exhaled from maximal inhalation to maximal exhalation

IL interleukin

JVP jugular venous pressure

LRTI lower respiratory tract infection

LTOT long-term oxygen treatment

MDI metered dose inhaler

NE neutrophil elastase

NOTT Nocturnal Oxygen Therapy Trial

NRT nicotine replacement therapy

NSAID non-steroidal anti-inflammatory drug

OSA obstructive sleep apnoea

Paco$_2$ arterial carbon dioxide tension

Pao$_2$ arterial oxygen tension

PDE phosphodiesterase

PEF peak expiratory flow – the maximal flow rate that can be maintained over the first 10 milliseconds of a forced blow

RV residual (lung) volume

TLC total lung capacity

TLco diffusing capacity for carbon monoxide, or diffusing capacity

TNF tumour necrosis factor

VC (relaxed or slow) vital capacity

1 Introduction

Main points

1 COPD is a common and important respiratory disorder that causes considerable morbidity and patient suffering.

2 It comprises a spectrum of diseases, including chronic bronchitis, emphysema, long-standing irreversible asthma and small airways disease.

3 COPD is a chronic, slowly progressive disorder characterised by airflow obstruction that varies very little from month to month.

4 The main cause of COPD is cigarette smoking.

5 COPD is more common in men and with increasing age. The prevalence is 2% of men aged 45–65 and 7% of men over 75 years. Some 26,000 people die from COPD each year in England and Wales.

6 It results in a large economic burden to the nation in excess of £500 million per year for health care.

7 The symptoms of breathlessness and coughing increasingly affect levels of activity, work, lifestyle and social interaction.

8 A co-ordinated approach for primary care, as set out in the British Thoracic Society's *COPD Guidelines*, will encourage the correct diagnosis, improve symptoms and quality of life, and prevent further deterioration.

Why COPD is important

Chronic obstructive pulmonary disease (COPD) is one of the most common and important respiratory disorders in primary care. About 26,000 people die from COPD each year in England and Wales, and the disease results in considerable morbidity, impaired quality of life, time off work, and more hospital admissions and GP consultations than asthma. However, its diagnosis and effective management have been largely neglected, apart from patients being advised to stop smoking.

COPD is a spectrum of diseases that includes:

■ chronic bronchitis,

■ small airways disease,

■ emphysema,

■ long-standing asthma that has become unresponsive to treatment.

The unifying feature of COPD is that it is a chronic, slowly progressive disorder characterised by airflow obstruction that varies very little from day to day and month to month.

COPD is caused mainly by cigarette smoking. However, only 20% of smokers will develop COPD and there are no clear pointers to what makes them particularly susceptible to the adverse effects of tobacco smoke. For people who are affected, stopping smoking is the only way to slow the progression of the disease. There are as yet no drugs that significantly improve the disease or alter the rate of decline of lung function.

The 1990s saw great improvements in the management and organisation of asthma treatment in primary care. COPD, by contrast, has been largely ignored and rightly has been dubbed the 'Cinderella respiratory disorder'. This situation began to change with the publication and widespread dissemination to GPs and practice nurses of the British Thoracic Society (BTS) *COPD Guidelines* in December 1997. Since then there has been considerable interest in the disease and its management. Research papers on COPD have flourished at both British and international meetings. The BTS Guidelines have set out five goals for COPD management:

■ early and accurate diagnosis,

- best control of symptoms,
- prevention of deterioration,
- prevention of complications,
- improved quality of life.

The present level of interest in COPD management is probably similar to that for asthma in 1990. The encouraging uptake of suggestions incorporated in the BTS Guidelines, together with an upsurge in training courses and postgraduate meetings, points to a much more rapid improvement in diagnosis and care than occurred with asthma in the early 1990s.

How important is COPD?

The Fourth National Morbidity Study published in 1992 calculated that there are about 600,000 people in the UK with diagnosed COPD – an overall prevalence of around 1%. Men are more likely to be affected than women, with prevalence rates of 2% in men aged 45–65 years and 7% in men over 75. The rates for women are rising, however, which is probably related to their increased smoking over the last 20 years. These figures are likely to be an under-estimate of the true prevalence, because much COPD may be mis-labelled as asthma. Moreover, most mild COPD goes unrecognised because patients are relatively asymptomatic, with only minor symptoms such as a smoker's cough or mild breathlessness on exertion. As a result, they often don't consult their doctor.

In 1994, COPD accounted for 5.4% of all deaths among men and 3.2% among women in the UK. Mortality tends to be greater in urban areas, particularly in South Wales, the north-west of England and Scotland. There is a strong association with lower social class and poverty that can be explained only partly by the higher smoking rates of this group.

A project for the future – when suitable government funding is made available – might be to screen smokers over the age of 45 years with spirometry (see Chapter 4) to detect early airflow obstruction before symptoms start. It will still be difficult to persuade people at risk to stop smoking but, if they are successful at this point of the disease, most of them will never develop symptomatic COPD. This will produce major personal benefits for them as well as a significant cost saving to the NHS.

As the disease progresses, patients become increasingly short of breath – washing, getting dressed and minimal exertion become difficult. The effect on lifestyle can be devastating, resulting in physical suffering, mood change and depression, together with social isolation. Many sufferers will have to accept early retirement, which can create financial problems for them. Even at a less severe level, many activities are restricted:

■ doing jobs around the house,

■ hobbies (e.g. gardening),

■ choice of holiday venues.

When one partner is significantly restricted, a marriage may be put under considerable strain.

An important part of COPD management is to be aware of these problems. Addressing social and psychological needs as well as encouraging patients to take as much regular exercise as possible should form an integral part of their care. Information on disability grants and aids, such as the Blue (formerly Orange) Badge parking scheme for people with disabilities, may help improve their overall quality of life.

What is the economic burden of COPD?

The total cost of COPD to the NHS is estimated to be £500 million a year. This sum is calculated from a primary care contribution of £262 million, which includes £85 million for prescriptions and £156 million for oxygen therapy. Secondary care adds £224 million, of which the major component is £174 million for emergency admissions.

A typical COPD patient consults 2.4 times per year, and has an estimated mean annual drug bill of £124. Oxygen therapy is an expensive part of treatment and the data suggest that oxygen is not being used most economically. About 30,000 patients with COPD receive oxygen therapy, and 23,000 of them use oxygen cylinders. The annual cost of regular use of oxygen by cylinder is £6,500 per patient, whereas the running costs of an oxygen concentrator are only £900 per year.

Patients with severe COPD often experience exacerbations of their symptoms – which are a common reason for their being admitted to hospital. In an average health district the annual inpatient bed days amount to 9,600, compared with 1,800 for asthma. The length of stay is notably longer than for asthma: 10 days for COPD compared with 3.6 days for asthma.

COPD also causes considerable loss of time from work – 21.9 million days in 1994. The economic cost for that period amounted to £331 million in state benefits. Adding the value of lost work to employers brings the total economic cost to the nation to a staggering £1.5 billion!

What can be done?

GPs and practice nurses can considerably improve the symptoms and lifestyle of patients with this very common disease. By making a correct diagnosis as early in the disease process as possible, maximum influence can be brought to bear on the patient to stop smoking and thus prevent the development of severe and disabling symptoms.

Once the disease is manifest, patients should be given the opportunity to have optimal bronchodilator therapy – the most important treatment to improve breathlessness and exercise tolerance. They need to be encouraged to exercise fully and to modify lifestyle factors, such as being overweight. The adverse social and psychological effects of the disease need to be recognised, carefully assessed and, where possible, alleviated. Patients with more severe disease may need to be referred to hospital for assessment for long-term oxygen, bronchodilators via nebuliser or possible surgery.

In the past the approach to managing COPD has been too negative. Much can be done for these patients, and primary care is the main site for their diagnosis and treatment. This book aims to equip you, as a primary care professional, to achieve this.

2 | Pathology and pathophysiology

Main points

1 COPD is not a discrete clinical entity, but a combination of chronic asthma, chronic bronchitis, small airway disease and emphysema.

2 The most important risk factor is cigarette smoking.

3 Treating persistent asthma early and aggressively with inhaled steroids may reduce the development of chronic airflow limitation.

4 Chronic mucus production alone is not always associated with the development of progressive airflow limitation; however, when there is progressive airflow limitation, chronic mucus production may accelerate the decline in lung function.

5 Emphysema is thought to develop as a result of an imbalance between elastase and anti-elastase activity in the lung.

6 Loss of lung elastin, such as occurs in emphysema, contributes to airway collapse, particularly during exercise.

7 Hyperinflation of the lungs leads to increased breathlessness on exertion.

8 Disruption of gas exchange leads to polycythaemia, cor pulmonale and respiratory failure.

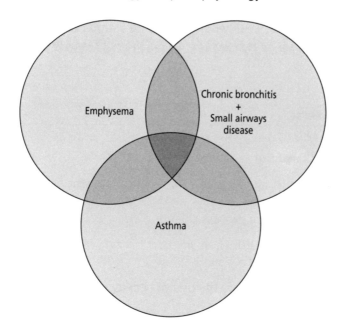

Figure 2.1 Diagrammatic representation of the four main conditions that comprise COPD

COPD is not a single disease entity, but comprises four main conditions (Figure 2.1):

- emphysema,
- chronic bronchitis,
- small airways disease,
- chronic asthma.

It has thus defied definition in terms of pathology, and the current definition of the British Thoracic Society is a functional one:

'a chronic, slowly progressive disorder characterised by progressive airflow obstruction (reduced FEV_1 and FEV_1/FVC ratio) that does not change markedly over several months.'

(FVC and FEV_1 are explained in Chapter 4.)

Some patients have an asthmatic element to their COPD and it will be possible to reverse their airflow obstruction to some degree. However, even when there is an asthma element, the lung function *cannot be returned to normal*, no matter how intensive the treatment.

Risk factors

Cigarette smoking

The most important risk factor for the development of COPD is cigarette smoking. Lung function declines after the age of 30–35 years as part of the ageing process (Figure 2.2).

- In normal, healthy non-smokers the rate of decline of FEV_1 is about 25–30ml a year.

- In 'at-risk' smokers the rate of decline may be double that, at about 50–60ml a year.

Why some smokers are at risk of this accelerated decline and others are not has been the subject of considerable research, but the answer remains elusive. Lung function declines steadily over the years of smoking but the FEV_1 often drops below 50% of predicted

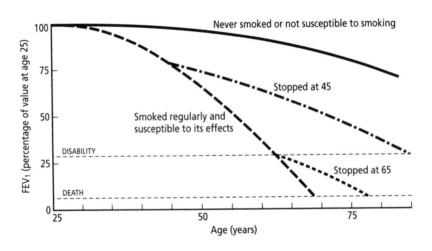

Figure 2.2 The decline in lung function as part of the normal ageing process and as accelerated by cigarette smoking.
(Reproduced, with permission, from Fletcher and Peto, 1977)

before symptoms appear. Patients usually present with symptoms of COPD between the ages of 50 and 70 years.

Although lost lung function is not regained when smoking is stopped, the rate of decline returns to that of a non-smoker or non-susceptible smoker. This highlights the importance of the early detection of such high-risk smokers and persuading them to stop smoking. If they can be persuaded to stop, they may never suffer from severe, disabling and symptomatic COPD.

Even when a smoker has developed symptomatic disease, stopping smoking will still result in worthwhile salvage of lung function and improved life expectancy. The main message for patients is:

It is never too late to stop!

Increasing age

COPD is a slowly progressive disorder, so increasing age is another risk factor. Symptoms appearing in someone under the age of 40 years should be regarded with suspicion and investigated fully because COPD is unlikely to be the cause, unless the sufferer is deficient in alpha-1 antitrypsin (α_1-AT). This is discussed in more detail later.

Gender

COPD is more common in men than in women. A national study of ventilatory function in British adults in the mid-1980s found reductions in lung function in the following proportions of people aged 40–65 years:

- 18% of male smokers,
- 7% of male non-smokers,
- 14% of female smokers,
- 6% of female non-smokers.

These differences between male and female smokers might be related to the fact that in this age cohort smoking was more common in men than in women. With the increase in the number of women smokers, it is likely that this preponderance of males will have changed.

Airway hyper-responsiveness

Airway hyper-responsiveness (AHR) has been proposed as a risk factor for the development of COPD. Certainly AHR is not the sole preserve of the person with asthma. It has been demonstrated extensively in smokers. Smokers also have raised levels of IgE, the antibody associated with atopy and asthma.

This observation forms the basis of the so-called Dutch hypothesis. Some doctors in the Netherlands have long regarded COPD and asthma as two aspects of the same process, and believe that at-risk smokers share an 'allergic' constitution that, when combined with smoking, is expressed as COPD. However, this hypothesis is controversial and it has been argued that raised levels of IgE and increased AHR in COPD patients could be the *result* of smoking rather than a pre-existing factor.

Lower socio-economic status

The prevalence of COPD is highest among people in lower socio-economic groups. Smoking rates are higher in these groups, but this may not be the sole causative factor.

Low birth weight is associated with a reduced FEV_1 in adult life. Airways develop in the first 16 weeks of gestation, and alveoli mature and increase in number in the last six weeks of gestation and first three years of life. The number of alveoli reaches adult levels of about 300 million by the age of 8 years. Thus, malnutrition of the fetus and serious lower respiratory tract infection (LRTI) in infancy during these periods of lung development may result in lung function failing to reach full potential. This may be an independent risk factor for reduced lung function in adult life and increased risk of COPD.

Maternal smoking has been extensively linked with low birth weight and recurrent LRTI in infancy, as have poor housing and social deprivation.

Poor diet

It has been suggested that antioxidants in the diet protect against the harmful effects of smoking and that a low dietary intake of antioxidant vitamins, such as vitamin C, is associated with decreased lung function and increased risk of COPD. Poor diet is also associated with socio-economic deprivation.

Occupation

Certain jobs have been linked with COPD. Coal mining is probably the most well-recognised occupational risk factor, but cotton processing, farming and other dusty occupations may also be relevant. Welding fumes are highly toxic, and welding, particularly in confined spaces, is suspected of being a risk factor. However, at present the only occupational cause of COPD for which compensation may be paid is coal mining.

Air pollution

Air pollution is often blamed by COPD sufferers for their disease. Before the Clean Air Acts of the 1950s, urban dwelling was associated with an increased risk: the air was polluted with heavy particles, soot and sulphur oxides. The pollution now experienced is mainly from vehicle exhaust emissions and photochemical pollutants such as ozone, produced by the action of sunlight on exhaust fumes. It is seldom disputed that these are respiratory irritants and that episodes of high pollution are associated with increased hospital admissions for respiratory problems. The role of these irritants *as a cause* of COPD, however, is more controversial. Nowadays, urban dwelling in the UK does not seem to pose a greater risk of COPD than rural dwelling.

Deficiency of alpha-1 antitrypsin

A rare, but well-recognised, risk factor for COPD is the inherited deficiency of alpha-1 antitrypsin. This is a protective enzyme that counteracts the destructive action of proteolytic enzymes in the lung. Deficiency of it is associated with the early development – between the ages of 20 and 40 years – of severe emphysema (see also the section 'Emphysema', below). The deficiency is inherited in a homozygous fashion with a frequency of 1:4,000 of the population. Both parents will be carriers but the possession of a single abnormal chromosome does not seem to cause severe disease. There is usually a strong family history of COPD. Family members should be tested for alpha-1 antitrypsin deficiency and, if affected, must be very strongly advised never to smoke.

Chronic asthma

Asthma is defined as:

> 'A chronic inflammatory condition of the airways, leading to widespread, variable airways obstruction that is reversible spontaneously or with treatment.'

Long-standing asthma may result in permanent damage to the airways and subsequent loss of that reversibility. Long-standing bronchial hyper-reactivity can cause hypertrophy of the bronchial smooth muscle, just as skeletal muscles will hypertrophy if exercised regularly. Chronic epithelial disruption may result in the deposition of collagen in the basement membrane and fibrosis of the submucosal layer. The end result is a narrowed and distorted airway that can no longer bronchodilate fully.

The duration and severity of the asthma are risk factors for the development of fixed airflow obstruction. Approximately 1 in 10 people with early-onset asthma will develop a degree of fixed airflow obstruction; for those with late-onset asthma the proportion is higher – around 1 in 4. Smoking considerably increases this risk.

Recent studies have suggested that early intervention with inhaled steroids reduces the risk. Work in children with persistent asthma has shown that a two-year delay in introducing inhaled steroids results in a reduced potential for the lung function to improve, compared with the improvement found in children who commenced inhaled steroids immediately. Further work with adults has shown similar results, suggesting that early diagnosis and early, aggressive treatment with inhaled steroids may reduce the risk of long-term chronic airflow obstruction. There are also implications for ensuring that patients adhere to the therapy they are prescribed and don't smoke.

Chronic bronchitis

Chronic bronchitis is defined by the Medical Research Council as:

> 'The production of sputum on most days for at least three months in at least two consecutive years.'

This definition describes a set of symptoms that are extremely common, if not universal, among long-term smokers and widely recognised as the 'smoker's cough'. Not all smokers whose illness fits the definition of chronic bronchitis will have an accelerated decline in lung function; 80% of smokers do not, after all, develop COPD. This chronic hypersecretion of mucus with little airflow obstruction is known as 'simple bronchitis'.

Mucus in the airways is produced by mucus glands, situated mainly in the larger airways, and by goblet cells, found mainly in the lining of the smaller airways. Mucus glands produce about 40 times more mucus than the goblet cells, and it may be that the excess mucus production in smokers not affected by progressive airflow obstruction reflects changes in the large airways. However, in at-risk smokers who are developing chronic airflow obstruction, excess mucus production seems to accelerate the rate of decline of their lung function.

Chronic production of mucus is unpleasant and may predispose the sufferer to lower respiratory tract infection, but on its own is not thought to be universally associated with the development of airflow obstruction. Excess production of mucus ceases in the majority of smokers when they stop smoking, although an initial short-term increase is a common experience in smokers when they quit.

Emphysema

Emphysema is defined in structural and pathological terms as:

> 'A condition of the lung characterised by abnormal, permanent enlargement of the air spaces distal to the terminal bronchiole, accompanied by destruction of their walls.'

This definition describes a destructive process that is largely associated with cigarette smoking. Cigarette smoke is an irritant and results in low-grade inflammation of the airways and alveoli. Broncho-alveolar lavage of smokers' lungs reveals increased numbers of inflammatory cells, notably macrophages and neutrophils. These inflammatory cells produce elastases – proteolytic enzymes that destroy elastin, the protein that makes up lung tissue. In health, these enzymes are neutralised by anti-elastases, anti-proteolytic enzymes, the most widely studied of which is alpha-1 antitrypsin. Figures 2.3 and 2.4 show the histology of normal lung tissue and of emphysema.

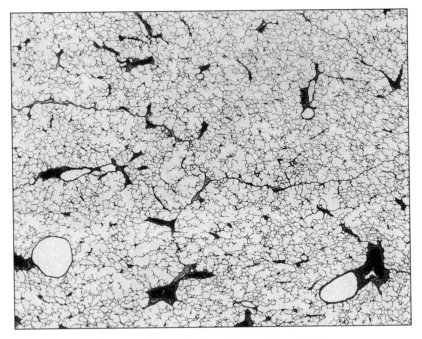

Figure 2.3 The histology of normal lung tissue

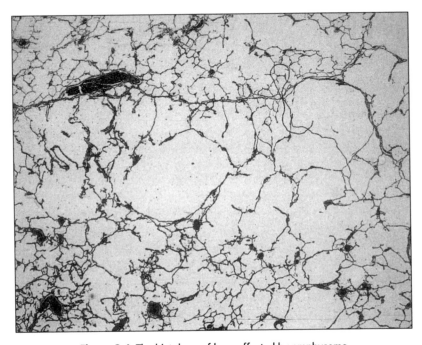

Figure 2.4 The histology of lung affected by emphysema

Alpha-1 antitrypsin deficiency accounts for 1–2% of all cases of diagnosed COPD. It provides a good model for our current understanding of the role of elastases and anti-elastases in the development of emphysema.

In early experiments, elastases introduced into lung tissue deficient in alpha-1 antitrypsin digested that lung tissue, thus producing emphysema. When alpha-1 antitrypsin was introduced into the deficient lung tissue – thereby effectively making it 'normal' – it protected against the action of the elastases and thus prevented emphysema.

That elastases are responsible for the destruction of lung tissue was confirmed by further experiments. A purified elastase was derived from neutrophils, a white blood cell attracted into the lungs of smokers. This neutrophil elastase (NE) was instilled into the lungs of experimental animals, causing a transient decrease in lung elastin, which then gradually returned to normal. However, although the loss of elastin was temporary, the structure of the animals' lungs was permanently damaged.

> The elastase/anti-elastase hypothesis for the development of emphysema in humans is that the irritant effect of cigarette smoke increases the level of elastases in the lungs beyond the body's ability to neutralise them. Over many years lung elastin is lost, lung tissue is destroyed and emphysema results.

Although these and other experiments helped to explain the mechanisms behind the development of emphysema in people who are deficient in alpha-1 antitrypsin, it remains less clear what happens in people who are not deficient in this anti-proteolytic enzyme. There are several theories but further investigation is needed.

One theory is that, in some smokers, excessive numbers of inflammatory cells are attracted into the lungs in response to the irritant effects of cigarette smoke. These inflammatory cells, particularly neutrophils, are responsible for the release of elastases into the lung tissue; if too many are attracted into the lung, the amount of elastase they produce may outstrip the protective capacity of the anti-elastases. It is thought that in some individuals the inflammatory cells themselves produce excessive amounts of elastases.

Yet another hypothesis is that there is excessive inactivation of the protective anti-elastases such that the individual is somewhat deficient in these protective enzymes. It is thought that this inactivation may be caused by oxidants that are both present in cigarette smoke and released from the activated inflammatory cells present in the airways of smokers.

These hypotheses can be summarised as:

- Abnormally high numbers of inflammatory cells are attracted into the airways, resulting in excessive production of elastases.

- The inflammatory cells in the airways produce abnormally large amounts of elastases.

- Oxidants found in cigarette smoke and released from inflammatory cells inactivate the protective anti-elastases in the lung.

In practice, all these mechanisms may be interacting in a single individual.

Elastases, NE in particular, have been implicated in the development of chronic bronchitis as well as emphysema. They have been found to produce an increase in the number of goblet cells, a feature of chronic bronchitis. NE is also a potent inducer of mucus secretion, and causes a reduction of ciliary beat frequency.

Thus elastase/anti-elastase imbalance may be implicated not only in the development of emphysema but also in the pathogenesis of chronic bronchitis.

Small airways disease

Cigarette smoking may result in pathological changes in the small airways as well as the alveoli. Structural changes in the small airways 2–5mm in diameter have been found in young smokers who have died suddenly from causes other than respiratory disease. The changes include:

- occlusion of the airway with mucus,

- goblet cell hyperplasia,

- inflammatory changes in the airway wall,

- fibrosis, and

- smooth muscle hypertrophy.

As a result, the airway becomes narrowed and distorted, causing resistance to airflow. Unfortunately, there can be considerable change in these airways without giving rise to symptoms. Indeed, this level of the bronchial tree is often referred to as the 'silent area' of the lungs.

COPD – a mixed spectrum of diseases

Although we can recognise the pathological entities of chronic bronchitis and emphysema, it is usual, clinically, for COPD patients to have features of both diseases.

Consequences

Narrowing of the bronchioles results in increased resistance to airflow. Loss of elastin in the alveolar walls in emphysema contributes to the collapse of the small airways. The lung parenchyma is made up of the walls of alveoli, which support the small airways in the same way that taut guy ropes hold open the walls of a tent. Destruction of the alveolar walls in emphysema means that this support is lost and the airways will tend to collapse (Figure 2.5). Airway collapse is exacerbated by forced exhalation, such as occurs on exercise, and air is trapped in the lungs. Patients with emphysema may naturally adopt a strategy that helps to 'splint' the airways open. 'Pursed-lip' breathing helps maintain air pressure in the small airways, preventing them from collapsing. Patients seem to be 'grabbing' air and 'paying it out' gently. It is a useful, though not universal, clinical sign.

The elastic walls of the alveoli provide some of the driving force behind exhalation. Loss of this elasticity causes the lungs to become 'floppy' and hyperinflated. Emphysematous lungs may be 2–3 litres bigger than normal, but most of this extra capacity is inaccessible.

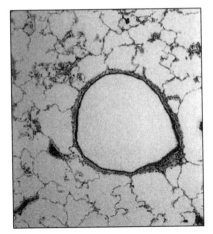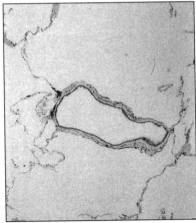

Figure 2.5 Histology showing the loss of the 'guy ropes', resulting in airway collapse

Hyperinflation causes the diaphragms to flatten and the accessory muscles of respiration are then used to aid respiration. The inefficient respiratory movements caused by hyperinflation lead to increased breathlessness on exertion, when the work of breathing is heightened and the respiratory rate is raised.

Loss of the alveolar/capillary interface causes disruption of gas exchange. The surface area for gas exchange in normal lungs is about the size of a tennis court. Emphysema reduces this area and thus reduces the capacity to exchange oxygen and carbon dioxide in the lungs. In the early stages of the disease the body is able to compensate for this loss by increasing the respiratory drive. As the disease progresses, however, the ability to compensate successfully diminishes and the blood gases become persistently abnormal, with serious consequences.

When the respiratory drive is responsive, abnormalities of blood gases will result in an increase in both respiratory drive and respiratory rate. The blood gases will be normalised but the patient will be breathless. Eventually the progression of the disease overcomes the ability of even the most responsive respiratory drive to compensate, and respiratory failure ensues.

Breathlessness makes everyday activities such as shopping, cooking and eating difficult. Weight loss is common and is associated with a poor prognosis. Although it was originally thought that weight loss in COPD was due to a combination of increased expenditure of energy at rest because of the increased effort of breathing and of difficulty in maintaining an adequate energy intake, it is now recognised that this is unlikely to be the sole cause. Loss of lean body mass affects the ability to fight infection. Infective exacerbations may become more common and recovery will be slower. (Weight loss and nutrition are discussed in more detail in Chapter 10.)

Some patients seem to have a less responsive respiratory drive and, as the disease progresses, they will become unable to normalise their blood gases. They will be less breathless but will suffer from the long-term consequences of low levels of oxygen in the blood (hypoxia), cor pulmonale, pulmonary hypertension and polycythaemia.

Cor pulmonale is a complex and incompletely understood syndrome of fluid retention and pulmonary hypertension caused by chronic **hypoxia**. The kidneys are affected by hypoxia, causing renin–angiotensin upset. This results in fluid retention and peripheral oedema.

Polycythaemia A way for the body to adapt to chronic hypoxia is to produce more haemoglobin to carry what little oxygen is available, increasing the number of erythrocytes and raising the packed cell volume (haematocrit). However, this predisposes an already less mobile patient to deep vein thrombosis and pulmonary embolism.

Pulmonary hypertension When areas of the lung are poorly ventilated – ventilation/perfusion mismatch – the alveolar capillary bed becomes constricted, causing increased pressure in the pulmonary vasculature – pulmonary hypertension. For a simplistic but helpful analogy for hypoxic pulmonary capillary constriction, imagine the lungs as a railway station. To work efficiently, passengers (*oxygen*) must reach the platforms (*alveoli*) where the trains (*blood supply*) can pick them up. If the passengers cannot reach the platforms (*poor ventilation*), the trains will go away empty and the railway system will be inefficient (*ventilation/perfusion mismatch*). If this situation persists, the railway line will be shut down (*pulmonary capillary constriction*). Eventually the track will be lifted so that, even if the passengers do reach the platform, the trains will no longer be there to pick them up. (Structural changes in the blood vessel walls eventually result in irreversible capillary constriction.)

The right ventricle has to work harder to pump an increased circulating volume of blood through a disrupted and constricted capillary bed. Initially it will enlarge to compensate for the extra workload, but will eventually fail, increasing the peripheral oedema. Clinically, cor pulmonale resembles right ventricular failure but, at least to begin with, the right ventricle may be functioning reasonably well.

The clinical pictures described above are recognisable as the 'pink puffer' and the 'blue bloater', but such terminology is currently out of favour and may not be particularly helpful. In practice the picture is less clear and patients often cannot be placed neatly into one or other category. Suffice it to say that some patients with appalling lung function and intolerable breathlessness will struggle on with reasonable blood gases whilst others, with less severely impaired lung function, will develop oedema and cor pulmonale relatively early. Intermittent ankle oedema and central cyanosis are a poor prognostic sign. Untreated, the three-year survival of such patients is only 30%. Long-term oxygen therapy (LTOT) can increase survival considerably; it is covered in detail in Chapter 10.

Further reading

Risk factors

AGERTOFT L, PEDERSEN S (1994) Effects of long-term treatment with an inhaled corticosteroid on growth and pulmonary function in asthmatic children. *Respiratory Medicine* **88**: 373–81

BARKER DJP, GODFREY KM, FALL C et al. (1991) Relation of birth weight and childhood respiratory infection to adult lung function and death from chronic obstructive lung disease. *British Medical Journal* **303**: 671–5

Cox BD (1987) Blood pressure and respiratory function. In: *The Health and Lifestyle Survey. Preliminary report of a nationwide survey of the physical and mental health, attitudes and lifestyle of a random sample of 9003 British adults.* Health Promotion Research Trust, London; 17–33

FLETCHER C, PETO R (1977) The natural history of chronic airflow obstruction. *British Medical Journal* **1**: 1645–8

HAAHTELA T, JARVINEN M, KAVA T et al. (1994) Effects of reducing or discontinuing inhaled budesonide in patients with mild asthma. *New England Journal of Medicine* **331**: 700–5

LEBOWITZ M (1977) Occupational exposures in relation to symptomatology and lung function in a community population. *Environmental Research* **44**: 59–67

LEBOWITZ MD (1996) Epidemiological studies of the respiratory effects of air pollution. *American Journal of Respiratory and Critical Care Medicine* **9**: 1029–54

MANN SL, WADSWORTH MEJ, COLLEY JRT (1992) Accumulation of factors influencing respiratory illness in members of a national birth cohort and their offspring. *Journal of Epidemiology and Community Health* **46**: 286–92

O'CONNOR GT, SPARROW D, WEISS ST (1989) The role of allergy and non-specific airway hyperresponsiveness in the pathogenesis of chronic obstructive pulmonary disease. *American Review of Respiratory Disease* **140**: 225–52

SCHWARTZ J, WEISS ST (1990) Dietary factors and their relation to respiratory symptoms. *American Journal of Epidemiology* **132**: 67–76

Pathology

MACNEE W (1995) Pulmonary circulation, cardiac function and fluid balance. In: Calverley P, Pride N (eds) *Chronic Obstructive Pulmonary Disease.* Chapman and Hall Medical, London; 243–91

PETO R, SPEIZER FE, MOORE CF et al. (1983) The relevance in adults of airflow obstruction, but not of mucous hypersecretion in mortality from chronic lung disease. *American Review of Respiratory Disease* **128**: 491–500

STOCKLEY RA (1995) Biochemical and cellular mechanisms. In: Calverley P, Pride N (eds) *Chronic Obstructive Pulmonary Disease.* Chapman and Hall Medical, London; 93–133

3 Presentation and history

Main points

1 COPD is rare in someone who has never smoked or is a genuinely light smoker.

2 A significant smoking history for COPD is more than 15–20 pack-years.

3 The commonest and most distressing symptom of COPD is breathlessness on exertion.

4 Symptoms are slowly progressive and non-variable.

5 COPD patients are generally not woken at night by their symptoms.

6 A previous history of asthma, atopic illness or childhood chestiness may point to a diagnosis of asthma rather than COPD.

7 Clinical signs of COPD are generally not apparent until the disease is severe.

8 Clinical signs in severe disease include:
- Barrel chest
- Prominent accessory muscles of respiration
- Recession of lower costal margins
- Abdominal breathing
- Weight loss
- Central cyanosis
- Peripheral oedema
- Raised jugular venous pressure

9 Alternative diagnoses must be carefully considered and excluded.

Symptoms

The most common presenting symptoms of COPD are breathlessness on exertion and cough, with or without sputum production. However, considerable loss of lung function can occur before symptoms become apparent, with the result that patients frequently consult their GP only when the disease is at an advanced stage. COPD is a slowly progressive disorder and patients gradually adapt their lives to their disability, not noticing breathlessness until it is severe enough to have a significant impact on their ability to perform everyday tasks. Most smokers expect to cough and be short of breath, and they often dismiss the symptoms of progressive airflow obstruction as a normal consequence of their smoking habit.

Breathlessness

The most important and common symptom in COPD, 'breathlessness' is a subjective term. It can be defined as an awareness of increased or inappropriate respiratory effort. Patients describe breathlessness in different ways, but the person with COPD will frequently describe it as difficulty inhaling:

'I just can't get enough air in!'

In health the increased oxygen demand that occurs with exercise is met by using some of the inspiratory reserve volume of the lungs to increase the tidal volume (see Figure 4.11). In COPD, because the calibre of the airways is relatively fixed, the inspiratory reserve volume cannot be fully used. Hyperinflation of the lungs with air-trapping in the alveoli leads to increased residual volume at the expense of inspiratory reserve volume, thus worsening breathlessness. Dynamic airway collapse due to loss of the 'guy ropes' (see Chapter 2) in emphysema causes further air-trapping, adding to the residual volume and increasing breathlessness on exertion. Flattening of the diaphragms when the lungs are hyperinflated means that the accessory muscles of respiration become increasingly important. Any activity, such as carrying shopping or stretching up, that uses these muscles for activities other than breathing will worsen breathlessness. COPD patients often also find it difficult to bend forward, for example to tie shoelaces.

Loss of the alveolar/capillary interface in COPD also means that the increased demand for oxygen that activity imposes cannot be met, and this also increases the sensation of breathlessness.

In asthma, breathlessness is variable; in COPD, it varies little from day to day. The answer to the question 'Do you have good days and bad days?' can thus be illuminating. The other major differences between the breathlessness of COPD and the breathlessness of asthma are that the patient with COPD is rarely woken at night by the symptoms and, until the disease is very severe, is not breathless at rest.

Although breathlessness is slowly progressive, patients will often relate the onset of symptoms to a recent event, notably a chest infection, and will claim to have 'Never been the same since then'. Close questioning will often reveal that the problem is indeed long-standing but that patients have unconsciously adapted their lifestyle to fit the disability. They will perhaps have avoided talking while walking, walked slower than their peers or have started to take the car when they would previously have walked. The chest infection was simply the 'straw that broke the camel's back'.

Cough

A productive cough either precedes or appears simultaneously with the onset of breathlessness in 75% of COPD patients. The cough is usually worse in the mornings but, unlike the asthma patient, the patient with COPD is seldom woken at night. Morning cough and chest tightness are usually quickly relieved by expectoration. Indeed, many patients justify the first cigarette of the day because it helps them to 'clear the tubes'. Morning symptoms in asthma frequently last for several hours.

Sputum

The production of sputum is a common, though not universal, feature of COPD. It is usually white or grey, but may become mucopurulent, green or yellow with exacerbations. It is generally less tenacious and 'tacky' than the sputum in asthma. Excessive production (half a cup full or more) of sputum and frequent infective episodes should raise the possibility of bronchiectasis, and any report of haemoptysis should be taken seriously. You should refer the patient immediately for chest x-ray and a consultant's opinion, because COPD patients have a high incidence of bronchial carcinoma.

The production of copious amounts of frothy sputum, particularly if it is associated with orthopnoea or a previous history of hypertension or ischaemic heart disease, may raise suspicions of left ventricular failure and pulmonary oedema.

Wheezing

Wheeze is a common presenting symptom in both COPD and asthma. COPD patients commonly experience wheeze when walking 'into the wind' or going out into cold air. Unlike people with asthma, they are rarely wheezy at rest and are not woken at night by wheeze. The atopic asthmatic will often relate wheezing episodes to exposure to a specific allergen.

History taking

COPD is unusual in a non-smoker, so it is important to quantify an individual's exposure to cigarettes as accurately as possible in terms of 'pack-years'. Smoking 20 cigarettes a day (a pack) for a year equates to one pack-year, 10 a day for a year is one-half pack-year, 40 a day for a year is two pack-years . . . and so on. The formula is:

$$\frac{\text{Number smoked per day}}{20} \times \text{Number of years smoked}$$

For example, if a patient smoked 10 cigarettes a day from the age of 14 years to 20 years, that is

$$\frac{10}{20} \times 6 = 3 \text{ pack-years}$$

When doing national service he started smoking seriously! – 20 a day until 45 years of age. That is:

$$\frac{20}{20} \times 25 = 25 \text{ pack-years}$$

Then he made a real effort to cut down and managed to get down to 5 a day until he finally stopped smoking aged 57 years:

$$\frac{5}{20} \times 12 = 3 \text{ pack-years}$$

It is therefore possible to calculate this patient's total cigarette exposure as

$$3 + 25 + 3 = 31 \text{ pack-years}.$$

A significant smoking history for COPD is more than 15–20 pack-years. If the smoking history is genuinely light, you should look carefully and exhaustively for other causes for the symptoms.

Any exposure to organic dusts, coal dust or welding fumes may be significant, so it is important to find out about a patient's occupational history. Bear in mind, too, that previous jobs might have exposed the patient to agents that could cause persistent, severe, occupational asthma.

It is important to establish when the symptoms started. 'Chestiness' in childhood might have been undiagnosed asthma that has recurred in adult life. Any family history of asthma or a previous history of atopic illness may point to a likelihood of asthma rather than COPD.

Smoking predisposes the patient to ischaemic heart disease as well as to COPD, and many older patients will be receiving treatment for hypertension. A full medical history and current drug therapy may highlight the possibility of a cardiac cause for the patient's symptoms.

Excluding other possible causes of breathlessness is very important. (Assessment and differential diagnosis are covered in detail in Chapters 4 and 5.)

Clinical signs

In mild and moderate disease, clinical signs are mostly absent. It is not until the disease is severe that clinical signs become apparent. *Early COPD is detectable only by measuring lung function with a spirometer.* (Spirometry is discussed in Chapter 4.) More can be gained by inspecting the chest than by examining it with a stethoscope. Removing the patient's shirt and taking a good look can be most informative. Although a definitive diagnosis does not depend on the examination alone, it is still an essential part of the assessment and can be used to support the history and the diagnostic tests. In severe disease the chest may be hyperinflated, with an increased anteroposterior diameter and a typical 'barrel' shape. The ribs become more horizontal and, because the position of the trachea is fixed by the mediastinum, the trachea may look shortened – the distance between the cricoid cartilage and the xiphisternal notch will be less than three finger-breadths. The trachea may also seem to be being pulled downwards with each breath.

Chest percussion may reveal that the liver is displaced downwards by the flattened diaphragms. Relatively quiet vesicular breath sounds may be heard on auscultation. Wheeze may also be audible, as may râles, particularly at the lung bases.

The strap muscles of the neck may be prominent and the lower intercostal margins drawn in on inhalation (Hoover's sign). Use of the abdominal muscles to aid exhalation may also be apparent, although movements of the rib cage during respiration may be relatively small. The angle between the lower ribs and the sternum – the xiphisternal angle – may widen because the ribcage is raised due to hyperinflation of the lungs. Flattening of the diaphragm may also displace the contents of the abdomen forward, giving the patient a pot-bellied appearance.

In severe disease the effort of walking into the consulting room and undressing will be sufficient to make most patients breathless, and the fact that breathing is hard work will be immediately obvious. They may lean forward, shoulders raised, resting their arms on the table to ease their breathing. Their respiratory rate will be raised and they may use 'pursed-lip' breathing. Their speech may be somewhat 'staccato' because they will not be able to complete a sentence without stopping for breath, and exhalation may be prolonged.

In patients with cor pulmonale the jugular venous pressure (JVP) will be raised, and there will be ankle oedema and central cyanosis. All of these are poor prognostic signs and must be taken seriously. Abnormal blood gases may be associated with loss of mental agility and the ability to concentrate. Elevated carbon dioxide may cause drowsiness and mental confusion, and a typical 'flapping' tremor of the hands when the arms are outstretched.

Finger clubbing is not a feature of COPD but may suggest bronchiectasis or a pulmonary tumour. Weight loss is common in advanced COPD, and another poor prognostic sign. Because malignancy is also a cause of weight loss in this group of middle-aged to elderly smokers, this must be excluded.

Summary

COPD presents as a slowly progressive, non-variable disease that causes breathlessness on exertion and cough with or without the production of sputum. The disease eventually affects every aspect of a patient's life and causes significant disability and handicap. Generally, clinical signs are apparent only when the disease is advanced, and the detection of early disease relies on a high level of suspicion about respiratory symptoms in patients who smoke and the referral of such patients for spirometry.

Further reading

CALVERLEY PMA, GEOGOPOULOS D (1998) Chronic obstructive pulmonary disease: symptoms and signs. In: Postma DS, Siafakis NM (eds) *Management of Chronic Obstructive Pulmonary Disease. European Respiratory Monograph:* **3** (May): 6–24

PEARSON MG, CALVERLEY PMA (1995) Clinical and laboratory assessment. In: Calverley P, Pride N (eds) *Chronic Obstructive Pulmonary Disease.* Chapman and Hall Medical, London; 309–49

Spirometry and lung function tests

Main points

1 Spirometry measures airflow and lung volumes, and is the preferred lung function test in COPD.

2 The forced vital capacity (FVC) is the total volume of air that can be exhaled with maximum force, starting from maximum inhalation and continuing to maximum exhalation.

3 The forced expiratory volume in one second (FEV_1) is the amount of air that can be exhaled in the first second of a forced blow from maximum inhalation.

4 Both the FVC and the FEV_1 are expressed as volumes (in litres) and as a percentage of the predicted values. Predicted values have been determined from large population studies, and are dependent on age, height, gender and ethnicity.

5 The ratio of FEV_1 to FVC (FEV_1/FVC) is expressed as a percentage. Values of less than 70% indicate airflow obstruction.

6 In diseases that cause airflow obstruction the FEV_1 will be below 80% of the predicted value and the FEV_1/FVC ratio will be less than 70%. (In severe COPD the FVC may also be less than 80% of predicted.)

7 In restrictive lung diseases both the FEV_1 and the FVC will be below 80% of the predicted value but the FEV_1/FVC ratio will be normal or high.

8 The volume/time trace must be smooth, upward and free of irregularities. The graph must reach a plateau, demonstrating that the patient has blown to FVC.

9 The forced expiratory manoeuvre can also be presented as graphs of flow rate against volume – the flow/volume trace. They show airflow through small airways and can be useful in distinguishing between asthma and COPD. They are, however, more difficult to interpret and are not essential for use in primary care.

10 Further tests, such as a gas transfer test (TLco) and static lung volumes, are available in lung function laboratories, and may be helpful.

11 Training in the proper use and interpretation of spirometry is essential.

Measuring lung function to determine the presence and severity of airflow obstruction in COPD is as fundamental as measuring blood pressure to detect and monitor hypertension.

The preferred and recommended lung function test is spirometry, which provides indices not only of airflow but also of lung volume. Since the publication of the BTS *COPD Guidelines*, general practices have been encouraged to obtain a spirometer. To benefit fully from its use, both doctors and practice nurses need training to understand the blowing technique and the interpretation of results. An alternative to having a spirometer in the practice may be open access spirometry at the local respiratory unit.

Spirometry

What does it mean?

In simple terms, spirometry measures two parameters – **airflow** from fully inflated lungs and the **total volume** of air that can be exhaled from maximum inhalation to maximum exhalation, using maximum force to blow all the air out as hard and as fast as possible. In a healthy individual this forced expiratory manoeuvre can normally be completed in three to four seconds, but with increasing airflow obstruction it takes longer to push all the air out of the lungs. In severe COPD it may take up to 15 seconds.

The volume of air exhaled is plotted on a graph against the time taken to reach maximum exhalation. Volume is plotted on the x (vertical) axis, and time on the y (horizontal) axis. This is known as the volume/time trace. Three indices can be derived from this trace:

1 FEV_1 – the forced expired volume in the first second.

2 FVC – the total volume of air that can be exhaled from maximal inhalation to maximal exhalation (the forced vital capacity).

3 $FEV_1/FVC\%$ – the ratio of FEV_1 to FVC, expressed as a percentage.

The FEV_1 and FVC are expressed in absolute values in litres and also as a percentage of the predicted values for that individual, depending on their age, height, gender and ethnic origin. For example, the predicted (mean) level of FEV_1 for a 30-year-old white male 1.70 metres tall is 3.86 litres and for a 65-year-old woman 1.50 metres tall it is 1.7 litres, based on a European Respiratory Society population survey conducted in 1993. Readings 20% either side of the predicted value are considered to be within the normal range. Thus an FEV_1 or FVC over 80% of the predicted value is normal.

When the airways are normal, 70–85% of the total volume of air in the lungs (FVC) can be exhaled in the first second. In other words, the FEV_1 normally comprises 70–85% of the FVC; the ratio of the FEV_1 to the FVC (FEV_1/FVC) is 70–85%. This is calculated by dividing the patient's FEV_1 by their FVC and multiplying by 100. When airflow through the airways is obstructed, less air can be exhaled in the first second and the FEV_1/FVC ratio falls. Levels below 70% indicate airflow obstruction. Examples of calculating lung function are given in Table 4.1.

Table 4.1 Calculating lung function in normal and obstructed patterns

Normal	*Obstructed*
FEV_1 = 3.0 litres	FEV_1 = 1.8 litres
FVC = 4.0 litres	FVC = 3.8 litres
$FEV_1/FVC\% = \dfrac{3.0}{4.0} \times 100$	$FEV_1/FVC\% = \dfrac{1.8}{3.8} \times 100$
= 75%	= 47%

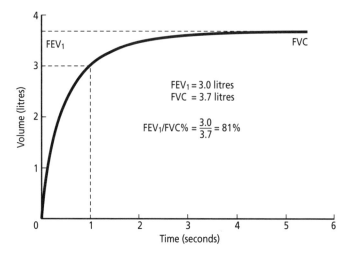

Figure 4.1 Normal spirometry (volume/time trace)

The shape of the volume/time trace should be smooth and convex upwards, and achieve a satisfactory plateau indicating that exhalation is complete (Figure 4.1). The FEV_1 is very reproducible and varies by less than 120ml between blows if the test is carried out correctly. The FVC can show more variation, as it will depend on

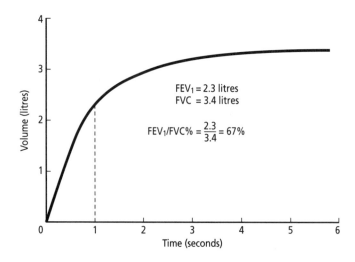

Figure 4.2 Mild obstruction

how hard the subject tries to blow the last remaining air out of the lungs.

Another extra manoeuvre, in addition to the forced expiratory manoeuvre discussed above, is the relaxed or slow vital capacity (VC), in which the patient blows out at their own pace after maximal inhalation. This can be useful in COPD when, because the airways may be unsupported, they might collapse during a forced blow. In COPD, the VC is often 0.5 litre greater than the FVC.

Obstructive pattern

With increasing airflow obstruction it takes longer to exhale and the early slope of the volume/time trace becomes less steep. Figures 4.2 and 4.3 show examples of mild and more severe obstruction. The FEV_1 is reduced both as a volume and as a percentage of the predicted value. The FEV_1/FVC likewise falls. The FVC in COPD and asthma is usually better maintained at near-normal levels until airflow obstruction is severe.

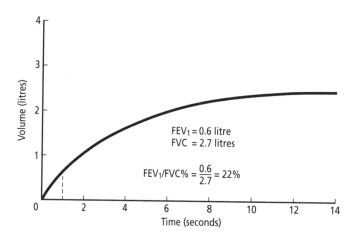

Figure 4.3 Severe obstruction

Restrictive pattern

Spirometry is helpful in the assessment of other respiratory conditions. In patients with, for example, lung scarring, diffuse fibrosis,

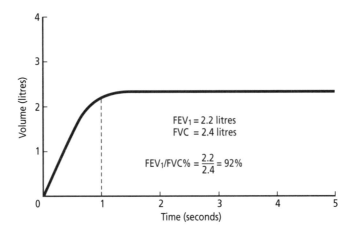

FEV$_1$ = 2.2 litres
FVC = 2.4 litres

FEV$_1$/FVC% = $\frac{2.2}{2.4}$ = 92%

Figure 4.4 Restrictive defect

pleural effusions or rib cage deformity the lung volumes become reduced. Airway size remains normal, which means that air can be blown out at the normal rate. This produces a trace (Figure 4.4) with a normal-shaped volume/time curve and a normal FEV$_1$/FVC ratio. The values of FEV$_1$ and FVC are reduced. This is called a restrictive pattern. Peak expiratory flow (PEF, see below) in such patients is normal.

Table 4.2 Summary of values for FEV$_1$, FVC, FEV$_1$/FVC ratio and PEF in normal, obstructive and restrictive patterns

	Normal	*Obstruction*	*Restriction*
FVC	above 80% predicted	above 80% predicted	below 80% predicted
FEV$_1$	above 80% predicted	below 80% predicted	below 80% predicted
FEV$_1$/FVC	above 70%	below 70%	above 70% (or high)
PEF	above 85% predicted	below 85% predicted	above 85% predicted

Table 4.3 Summary of likely conditions causing obstructive or restrictive disease

Obstructive disease	Restrictive disease
Generalised obstruction	Sarcoid
Asthma	Fibrosing alveolitis
COPD	Extrinsic allergic alveolitis
Bronchiectasis	Malignant infiltration
Cystic fibrosis	Asbestosis
Obliterative bronchiolitis	Pleural effusions
	Kyphoscoliosis
Localised obstruction	Ascites
Tumour	Obesity
Inhalation of foreign body	
Post-tracheotomy stenosis	

Table 4.2 summarises the values for FEV_1, FVC, FEV_1/FVC ratio and PEF in normal, obstructive and restrictive patterns. Table 4.3 categorises the conditions likely to be causing obstructive or restrictive disease.

Blowing technique and reproducibility

Preparing the patient

- The patient should be clinically stable (i.e. at least four weeks should have elapsed since the last exacerbation).
- The patient should not have taken any bronchodilator (no beta-agonist or anticholinergic inhaler) for six hours.
- The patient should not be wearing a corset or other restrictive clothing, and should remove any loose-fitting dentures or chewing gum.
- Ensure that the patient is comfortable; invite them to empty their bladder before proceeding.

Blowing technique

- The patient should be sitting in an upright position (not standing, because there is a potential risk of their feeling faint or dizzy, especially after repeated blows).

- Explain and demonstrate the technique to the patient.

- Ask the patient to take a maximal breath in and then place their lips around the mouthpiece to form an airtight seal.

- Ask the patient to exhale as hard, fast and completely as possible (with lots of encouragement from you). In a healthy person it may take only three to four seconds to complete the blow. With increasing airflow obstruction, it becomes harder to blow air out rapidly and exhalation can take as long as 15 seconds.

- Allow the patient adequate time – including time for recovery between blows, with a maximum of six forced manoeuvres in one session.

Technical standards

- Three technically satisfactory manoeuvres should be made, giving similar results (good reproducibility) (see Figure 4.5).

- The best two readings of FEV_1 should be within 100ml or 5% of each other.

Common faults

The most common faults are:

- stopping blowing too early,

- coughing during the blow,

- submaximal effort.

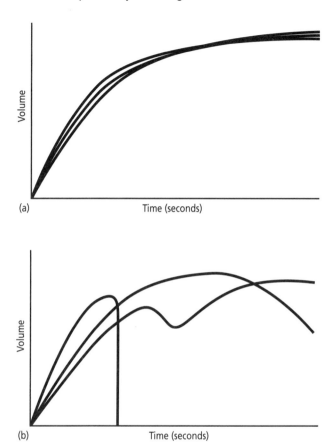

Figure 4.5 **(a)** Good reproducibility of blows; **(b)** poor reproducibility

Why is FEV_1 the preferred test?

The British, American, European and other national COPD guidelines all use FEV_1 as a percentage of predicted value as the basis for diagnosis and for estimating the severity of the disease. The BTS *COPD Guidelines* use the following scale:

- FEV_1 % predicted 60–80% – mild disease,
- FEV_1 % predicted 40–59% – moderate disease,
- FEV_1 % predicted below 40% – severe disease.

The FEV_1 is the measurement of choice because:

- It is reproducible with well-defined normal ranges according to age, height and gender.

- It is quick and relatively easy to measure.

- Other diagnostic measurements such as FVC and FEV_1/FVC are recorded, which help in differential diagnosis.

- Variance of repeated measurements in any individual is low.

- FEV_1 predicts future mortality not only from COPD but also from other respiratory and cardiac disorders.

- FEV_1 is better related to prognosis and disability than FEV_1/FVC; this is mainly because the FVC, depending as it does on effort, is more variable.

The peak expiratory flow (PEF) measures the maximal flow rate that can be maintained over the first 10 milliseconds (ms) of a forced blow. It often under-estimates the degree of airflow obstruction in COPD, and the relationship between PEF and FEV_1 is poor in COPD. (In asthma the correlation is better.)

Types of spirometer

Spirometers are essentially of two types:

- they measure volume directly (e.g. the dry bellows type of device),

- they measure flow through a pneumotachograph and electronically convert the values into volumes.

Electronic spirometers, which are mostly of the second type, usually have the facility to enter patient's age, height and gender, and will automatically calculate predicted values and the percentage of normal of the measured values. They have real-time traces of each blow, which can be superimposed on each other and the variance calculated to assist in assessing reproducibility. Many will also produce a flow/volume curve (see below) as well as the volume/time trace.

There are many effective spirometers, from the simple hand-held electronic device costing about £300 to more sophisticated equipment with many other facilities which can cost up to ten times that amount. Primary care needs are for simple, easy-to-use spirometers that preferably produce a hard copy printout of the trace and results. Some spirometers offer the facility for results and traces to be stored on a computer database. This type of equipment usually costs at least £1300. The low-cost hand-held devices do not allow a proper assessment of the quality or reproducibility of the procedure.

Nearly all spirometers require regular calibration with a 3-litre syringe but the manufacturers of some electronic devices claim that their instrument is accurate for at least three years without further calibration.

Training in the use of the spirometer and in the interpretation of results is essential. Courses for doctors and nurses are becoming increasingly available from official nurse training centres such as the National Asthma and Respiratory Training Centre (NARTC) and from spirometer manufacturers. Training may also be available at local lung function centres.

Lung age

Some electronic spirometers will calculate 'lung age' from the measured and predicted FEV_1. If the FEV_1 is reduced, this factor may be used to try to persuade patients to stop smoking – for example, knowing that their lung age is, say, 10–15 years greater than their actual age can be a powerful incentive.

Flow/volume measurement

Many modern spirometers measure a plot of expiratory flow rate throughout the entire expiratory blow, at the same time as the standard volume/time trace. A PEF, in contrast, measures only the maximal flow rate that can be sustained for 10 milliseconds and represents flow only from the larger airways. The flow/volume trace, on the other hand, interprets flow from all generations of airways and is more helpful in detecting early narrowing in small airways, as in early COPD. It is also useful for differentiating between asthma and COPD, and can help to determine when there are mixed obstructive and restrictive defects.

For primary care purposes, interpretation need only extend to understanding the shape of the flow/volume curve. Figures 4.6, 4.7

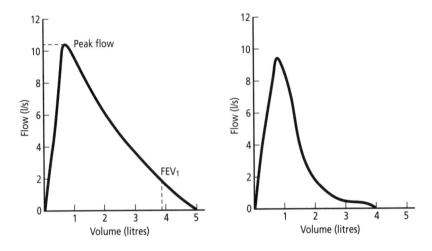

Figure 4.6 Normal flow/volume curve   **Figure 4.7** Mild obstruction

and 4.8 give examples of normal, mild and moderate airflow obstruction. Figure 4.9 shows the classic 'steeple' pattern of airway collapse with emphysema, in which airways suddenly shut down on forced exhalation with low residual flow from the smaller airways.

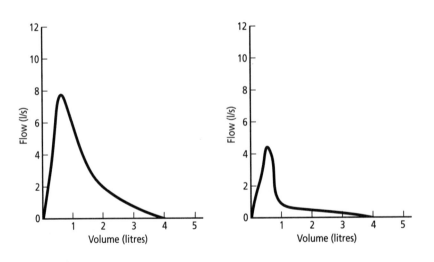

Figure 4.8 Moderate obstruction   **Figure 4.9** 'Steeple' tracing in severe emphysema

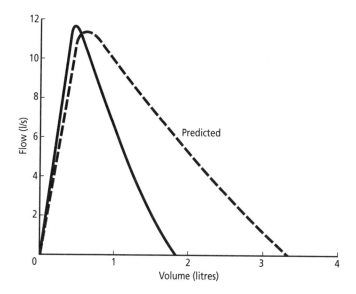

Figure 4.10 Restrictive pattern

Figure 4.10 demonstrates the restrictive pattern with a normal shape curve and PEF but small FVC.

Other uses of spirometry

Measuring FEV_1 and FVC provides much more information than a simple PEF. Spirometers can therefore be useful in screening and following a whole range of respiratory disorders. The main areas of use are:

■ obstructive lung disease,

■ restrictive lung diseases,

■ diagnosing and monitoring occupational lung disease,

■ screening of smokers,

■ medical examinations for scuba diving, aviation and insurance,

■ health screening and possible screening of new patients (although the value of screening in asymptomatic non-smokers is controversial).

Early screening for COPD

In an ideal world, there might be advantages to screening populations at risk – smokers from about 40 years onwards – to detect early indications of airflow obstruction. This could be enhanced with a flow/volume trace, which is the most sensitive simple test for detecting early changes. Stopping patients smoking at this stage – admittedly not an easy task – would largely prevent COPD in most of them as well as reducing their risk of lung cancer and cardiovascular disease. In the long term there could be considerable cost saving for the nation. Unfortunately, there are not the money, time, resources and staff available to perform widespread screening at present.

Peak expiratory flow (PEF)

PEF is a simple, quick and inexpensive way of measuring airflow obstruction. It has been particularly useful in the diagnosis and monitoring of asthma.

The PEF meter measures the maximal flow rate that can be maintained over 10 milliseconds and usually detects a narrowing of large and medium-sized airways. It is most effective for monitoring changes in airflow in an individual over time. It has less value diagnostically because, as mentioned earlier, it may under-diagnose the severity of airflow obstruction in COPD.

The blowing technique requires the patient to inhale fully and then make a short maximal blow into the device (likened to blowing out candles on a birthday cake). The reading is expressed in litres per minute (l/min). It should be noted that, because the expiratory blowing technique is quite different from that required for spirometry, the readings for PEF will not be the same as those obtained from a peak flow meter. The reading from a PEF meter is usually greater by 50–100 litres per minute. The result from blowing into a PEF meter is less reproducible than with spirometry, and some patients use some very strange techniques for blowing – from a cough-like action to almost spitting into the device.

PEF can be helpful in COPD but should never be considered diagnostic or quantitative in terms of severity. It can be useful to perform twice-daily readings at home during a trial of an oral steroid or when it is uncertain whether the diagnosis is asthma or COPD.

Gas transfer test (TLco)

This very useful test is performed in hospital lung-function laboratories. The single-breath diffusion test measures the ability of the alveolar air/blood interface to transfer a trace amount of carbon monoxide into the pulmonary circulation. A number of factors affect it, of which the main ones are:

- the thickness and amount of the alveolar membrane,

- the capillary blood volume,

- the haemoglobin concentration (the test needs to be corrected for haemoglobin level).

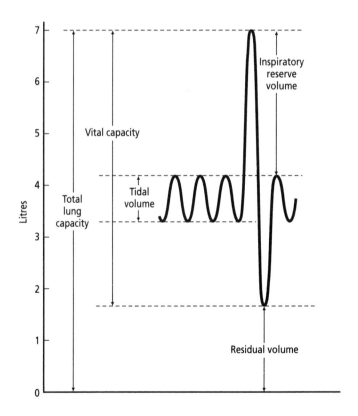

Figure 4.11 Lung volumes

Gas transfer is significantly reduced in more severe degrees of emphysema, because of the loss of alveolar tissue. (Gas transfer is also reduced in fibrosing alveolitis, allergic alveolitis and other causes of diffuse fibrosis.) In asthma, gas transfer is normal.

Static lung volumes (Figure 4.11)

Measurement of the total lung capacity (TLC) and residual volume (RV) using a body plethysmograph apparatus is occasionally used in hospital when assessing patients for lung surgery for COPD. In emphysema, residual volume is greatly increased because of the volume of air trapped in enlarged air sacs and by airway collapse due to loss of the 'guy ropes' effect (see Chapter 2).

CT lung scans in inhalation and exhalation can also be used to measure lung volumes.

5 Assessment

Main points

1 Bronchodilator reversibility tests should be performed, using high doses of both beta-agonists and anticholinergics.

2 Corticosteroid reversibility tests should be tried in all patients who present with moderate or severe disease, and in patients with mild disease who need to use a bronchodilator more than once a day to relieve symptoms.

3 Tests of reversibility both to bronchodilators and to corticosteroids must be performed during a period of clinical stability.

4 A positive result is an increase in FEV_1 that is greater than 200ml and 15% over baseline.

5 A negative bronchodilator reversibility test does not mean that the patient will not benefit from long-term bronchodilators; therapeutic trials of several weeks' treatment should be undertaken.

6 In patients presenting with severe disease, a referral for arterial blood gases may be indicated, especially if there are signs of cyanosis, raised jugular venous pressure, peripheral oedema or polycythaemia.

7 Other possible causes of the patient's symptoms must be considered and excluded.

8 Formal assessments of disability and handicap should be performed as a baseline from which to assess the effectiveness of any treatment.

Making the diagnosis and establishing a baseline

Spirometry is essential to the diagnosis of COPD, and is discussed in Chapter 4. Nevertheless, although it is a crucial aid to the diagnosis of airway obstruction, spirometry is unable to determine its cause. A full history (discussed in Chapter 3) and tests of reversibility are also needed. The history, signs and symptoms may suggest a diagnosis of COPD but cannot confirm it. Neither can they define the treatment or the prognosis. By definition, COPD is irreversible airflow obstruction, so exhaustive tests must be undertaken to ensure that reversibility is not missed.

Bronchodilator reversibility

The two main objectives of bronchodilator reversibility testing in COPD are:

- To detect patients who have a substantial increase in the FEV_1, and are therefore suffering from asthma.

- To establish the post-bronchodilator FEV_1, the best predictor of long-term prognosis.

The testing should be performed regardless of the stage of the disease at presentation. Even people with severe airflow obstruction can achieve reversibility.

Reversibility tests must be conducted during a period of clinical stability when the patient is free of infection. Because small doses of bronchodilator will produce a response in fewer people, high doses of bronchodilator should be used in order not to miss a significant response. The most convenient way to deliver high-dose bronchodilators reliably is via a nebuliser. An alternative method is to deliver a similar dose of drug by giving repeated doses from a metered dose inhaler (MDI) via a large volume spacer.

The British Thoracic Society's suggested protocol for testing bronchodilator reversibility is:

- Record FEV_1 before and 15 minutes after giving 2.5–5mg nebulised salbutamol or 5–10mg nebulised terbutaline.

- Record (preferably on a separate occasion) FEV_1 before and 30 minutes after 500μg nebulised ipratropium bromide or

■ Record FEV_1 before and 30 minutes after a combination of
  salbutamol (or terbutaline) and ipratropium.

*An increase in the FEV_1 that is both greater than 200ml and 15% over
the baseline is interpreted as a positive result.* Patients whose
improvement is greater than this have a significant degree of
reversibility, and an early corticosteroid reversibility test is
indicated.

Even when there is no significant reversibility to bronchodilators
on formal testing, patients with COPD may still benefit from long-
term bronchodilator therapy in terms of improved functional ability
and well-being or decreased breathlessness. It is thought that, in the
longer term, bronchodilators reduce air-trapping and over-inflation
of the lungs, thus improving both respiratory muscle mechanics and
exercise tolerance and breathlessness. Trials of several weeks of
treatment with different drugs, different combinations of drugs and
different doses are needed to establish which is the most effective
treatment for each individual, even when the reversibility tests have
proved negative. The use of bronchodilators in COPD is discussed
in Chapter 7.

The measures of outcome from therapeutic trials of bronchodilators in COPD are different from those used in the diagnostic
reversibility testing described above. Improvements in lung function
cannot be anticipated and should not be sought. Improvements in
functional ability and/or breathlessness are more significant. Methods of objectively measuring these rather subjective effects are
discussed in detail later in this chapter.

The post-bronchodilator FEV_1, as a percentage of the predicted
FEV_1, is used to classify the severity of COPD:

■ FEV_1 60–80% predicted   Mild disease

■ FEV_1 40–59% predicted   Moderate disease

■ FEV_1 below 40% predicted   Severe disease

The prognosis is also directly related to the post-bronchodilator
FEV_1 and inversely related to the patient's age. The post-bronchodilator value correlates better with survival than the pre-broncho-
dilator value:

■ Aged under 60
   and FEV$_1$ above 50% predicted   90% 3-year survival

■ Aged over 60
   and FEV$_1$ above 50% predicted   80% 3-year survival

■ Aged over 60
   and FEV$_1$ 40–49% predicted   75% 3-year survival

Corticosteroid reversibility

Reversibility to corticosteroids – steroid responsiveness – is shown in 10–20% of patients with clinically stable COPD. It is most likely in patients who have achieved significant reversibility in bronchodilator reversibility tests, but even those who have no bronchodilator reversibility can respond to a corticosteroid trial. (Steroid reversibility also helps identify potential asthmatics.)

As with bronchodilator reversibility tests, corticosteroid reversibility testing should be done during a period of clinical stability.

The BTS Guidelines recommend that prednisolone 30mg is given daily for two weeks. Spirometry is recorded before and immediately at the end of the trial. An alternative approach for patients who are unable to tolerate oral steroids is to give a six-week trial of inhaled corticosteroid, beclomethasone 1000μg per day, or equivalent.

The criteria for a positive response are the same as for bronchodilator reversibility testing: 200ml and 15% improvement in FEV$_1$ over baseline. A non-research-based alternative to spirometry suggested by the BTS is an improvement of 20% or more in the mean peak expiratory flow rate over the first and last five days of a trial. Some patients experience euphoria and a general feeling of well-being on oral corticosteroids. Current guidelines suggest, however, that such responses should not be taken as a positive result, and that only patients whose lung function improves should be treated with long-term inhaled steroids.

A corticosteroid reversibility test is probably not needed in mild COPD when the patient is using a bronchodilator only occasionally (not more than once a day). If, however, bronchodilators are needed more often than this to relieve symptoms, even if the post-bronchodilator FEV$_1$ is compatible with a diagnosis of mild COPD (i.e. between 60% and 80% predicted), a corticosteroid reversibility test should be performed. Tests should be carried out in all patients presenting with moderate to severe disease. Even those with severe disease can achieve reversibility, and it is important that they are not missed.

The role of corticosteroids in the long-term treatment of COPD remains controversial and is the subject of ongoing research. It is discussed further in Chapter 8.

Excluding alternative and coexisting pathologies

Lung cancer is an important differential diagnosis to consider. The incidence of lung cancer is high among patients with COPD, so any middle-aged or elderly smoker presenting with respiratory symptoms should have a chest x-ray to exclude this.

If the chest x-ray reveals 'emphysematous changes' or 'hyperinflation', this will add weight to a diagnosis of COPD, although hyperinflation may also be a feature of chronic asthma. Emphysema may be assessed by computed tomography (CT) – see Figure 5.1. CT can also be used in the diagnosis of bronchiectasis.

A chest x-ray may show bullous emphysema, which can be treated surgically. It may reveal cardiac enlargement and pulmonary oedema, prompting cardiac investigation.

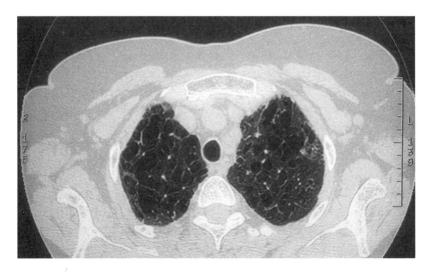

Figure 5.1 A CT scan, showing emphysema

The chest x-ray need not be repeated routinely, but an unexplained change in symptoms should be regarded with suspicion. Often the change in symptoms is reported by the patient's carer and is rather ill-defined and vague: 'He just hasn't been the same recently'. Such a history, failure of a chest infection to resolve or haemoptysis merits a repeat chest x-ray to exclude a tumour.

An electrocardiogram will help in the differential diagnosis of cardiac breathlessness, provided it is correctly interpreted. In some areas, there is open access to echocardiography. A review of the patient's current medication may also lend weight to a diagnosis of cardiac breathlessness or reveal the use of beta-blockade which may have precipitated asthma.

A full blood count should be taken to exclude anaemia as a cause of breathlessness. It will also reveal polycythaemia in the chronically hypoxic patient. A referral for arterial blood gases is indicated if:

- polycythaemia is present

or there are signs of:

- cor pulmonale,

- raised jugular venous pressure,

- central cyanosis,

- peripheral oedema.

Hypoxia and hypercapnia (raised levels of CO_2 in the blood) are common in severe COPD, and measurement of arterial blood gases should be considered for patients presenting with severe disease. Pulse oximetry, if there is access to it in the practice, may be a useful screening tool. If the oxygen saturation is over 92% and the patient is not deteriorating clinically, the measurement of arterial blood gases may not be necessary at that time.

Diseases that cause pulmonary fibrosis (e.g. fibrosing alveolitis) may present as breathlessness on exertion and may be confused with COPD. However, the spirometry will not reveal obstruction. The FEV_1 /FVC ratio will be normal or high but the lung volumes, the FEV_1 and the FVC will be low. Patients with this pattern of restricted spirometry require assessment by a respiratory physician and are generally beyond the scope of primary care management.

Severe obstructive sleep apnoea (OSA) can present as cor pulmonale. The upper airway obstructs during sleep, producing repeated apnoea sufficient to cause a significant drop in oxygen saturation levels and to rouse the sufferer repeatedly. Patients have a history of 'heroic' snoring and they complain of daytime somnolence. They may have a poor driving accident record because they fall asleep at the wheel. OSA is more common in men than women, and sufferers are often obese, with a collar size of 17 inches or more. Although OSA is an upper respiratory problem and is not related to COPD, it may coexist with it, particularly in patients who are overweight or Cushingoid due to long-term use of oral steroids.

Disability and handicap

Once it has been established that the patient has irreversible airflow obstruction and alternative diagnoses have been excluded, it is important to measure the impact of the disease on the patient's everyday life: the level of disability and handicap. These considerations are frequently overlooked, but it is these effects that are most important to the patient and are the areas that treatment of COPD aims to improve.

Because airways obstruction is largely fixed, big improvements in lung function are not attainable but improvements in disability and handicap are. For the patient such outcomes are far more important than, for example, an improvement of 100ml in the FEV_1, because they equate more with their ability to carry on their everyday lives. You will need a baseline level of disability and handicap from which to assess accurately the effectiveness of any intervention.

Assessing breathlessness

'Breathlessness' is a subjective feature, but it is important to quantify this because improvement in breathlessness is one of the most important ways of seeing whether treatment is working. There are several scales for assessing it objectively.

The MRC dyspnoea scale (Table 5.1) allows patients to rate their breathlessness according to the activity that induces it. It is graded from 0 to 5.

Whilst the MRC scale is helpful and easy to use, it is relatively insensitive to change and may be more valuable as a baseline assessment rather than as a tool for measuring the effect of a treatment.

Table 5.1 MRC dyspnoea scale

Grade	Degree of breathlessness related to activities
0	Not troubled by breathlessness except on strenuous exercise
1	Short of breath when hurrying or walking up a slight hill
2	Walks slower than contemporaries on the level because of breathlessness, or has to stop for breath when walking at own pace
3	Stops for breath after walking about 100m or after a few minutes on the level
4	Too breathless to leave the house, or breathless when dressing or undressing
5	Breathless at rest

The oxygen cost diagram is more sensitive to change than the MRC scale; it allows the patient to place a mark on a 10cm line, beyond which they become breathless (Figure 5.2). The ability score is the distance in centimetres from the zero point.

Other scales allow patients to grade their breathlessness according to the intensity of the sensation. The Borg scale (Table 5.2) is

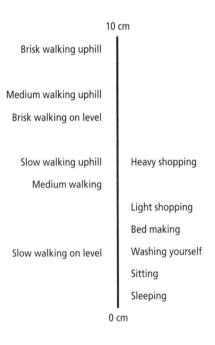

Figure 5.2 The 'oxygen cost' diagram

Table 5.2 The Borg scale

0	Nothing at all
0.5	Very, very slight (just noticeable)
1	Very slight
2	Slight (light)
3	Moderate
4	Somewhat severe
5	Severe (heavy)
6	
7	Very severe
8	
9	
10	Very, very severe (almost maximal) Maximal

useful for measuring short-term changes in the intensity of the breathlessness during a particular task. It is both sensitive and reproducible.

A simple visual analogue scale is another method of allowing patients to rate the intensity of their breathlessness. As with the oxygen cost diagram, a 10cm line is drawn on a page and the patient then marks on the line how intense their breathlessness is, from 0cm (nothing at all) to 10cm (intensely breathless). The score is the distance along the line that the patient has marked.

Assessing walking distance

A six-minute walking test and a shuttle walking test are also methods of objectively measuring disability. The six-minute walk measures the distance a patient can walk in six minutes, indoors, on the flat. The patient does a practice walk first, to give them confidence, and measurements are taken on the second walk. The patient is actively encouraged throughout, and stops for rest are allowed. In a shuttle test the patient performs a paced walk between two points 10 metres apart (a shuttle). The pace of the walk is increased at regular intervals, dictated by 'beeps' on a tape recording, until the patient is forced to stop because of breathlessness. The number of completed shuttles is then recorded.

If neither the six-minute walk nor the shuttle walking test is fea-
sible in the practice, you should ask the patient how far they are
able to walk; comparisons between walking distance before and
after any intervention can still be useful. Asking how many lamp
posts the patient can walk past before they get breathless, before
and after a given intervention, may be a practical way to assess
walking distance objectively in a primary care setting.

Impact of the disease on pychosocial functioning

Increasing disability and breathlessness on exertion eventually
affect all areas of the patient's psychological, sexual and social
functioning. An individual's perception of their health status is
closely associated with their personality and the amount of social
support they have; those with supportive families do better than
those who live alone. Some patients with relatively good lung
function may be significantly disabled, have given up work and be
isolated and depressed, whereas others with appalling lung function
may continue to work and remain active and cheerful.

Attacks of breathlessness frequently produce feelings of fear and
panic. Episodes in public can cause anxiety and embarrassment, and
the wish to avoid such feelings may well sow the seeds of social isolation. Depression is common, significantly affecting an individual's
ability to cope with the disease and lessening the effectiveness of
any therapeutic intervention. Treating coexisting depression can
have a very significant beneficial effect on the patient's health status
and overall quality of life.

Loss of independence frequently causes feelings of anger, frustration or resentment, often manifested as impatience with the
person closest to the patient. Such feelings result in loss of self-
esteem and may cause self-destructive behaviour, such as a refusal
to stop smoking. The way that patients often cope with these very
negative feelings is to withdraw physically and emotionally. Many
COPD patients live in an 'emotional straitjacket' (see Chapter 9).

Assessing health status

Assessing health status in COPD, like measuring breathlessness and
disability, is important because it too may be improved.

There are several questionnaires available for the measurement of health status, mostly used in hospital rehabilitation programmes and research. The Chronic Respiratory Disease Index Questionnaire is very sensitive to change, but is also the most cumbersome and time consuming to use, and requires training to administer properly. The St George's Respiratory Questionnaire, a 'self-fill' questionnaire is more practical but may be slightly less sensitive. Another 'self-fill' questionnaire is the Breathing Problems Questionnaire. This is user-friendly but relatively insensitive to change.

Such formal questionnaires are most useful in the setting of a formal rehabilitation programme. In general practice, a simple enquiry about the two or three most distressing daily activities may suffice. Include questions about the patient's overall feelings of fatigue and about their emotional state. Depression may manifest itself as panic, anxiety or feelings of helplessness and hopelessness.

The degree of control that a patient feels may be assessed by asking such questions as:

- 'How confident do you feel about dealing with your illness?'

- 'Do you feel upset or frightened by your attacks of breathlessness?'

- 'Do you feel in control of your breathlessness?'

- 'Do you feel tired?'

- 'Do you ever feel down?'

Summary

Middle-aged or elderly patients with respiratory symptoms, particularly those with a significant smoking history, pose a challenge to the health professional. There may have been a tendency to class all breathless smokers as suffering from COPD but it is extremely important not to become blinkered. Smokers are at risk of many other smoking-related diseases, such as ischaemic heart disease or lung cancer, and they may have other lung disease or coexisting pathologies that make assessment difficult. All patients deserve a thorough assessment to make sure that other pathologies are not missed and that appropriate treatment is given and its effectiveness properly assessed.

Further reading

Assessment of impairment

British Thoracic Society (1997) BTS guidelines for the management of chronic obstructive pulmonary disease. *Thorax* **52** (Suppl 5): S1–S28

BURROWS B (1991) Predictors of cause and prognosis of obstructive lung disease. *European Respiratory Review* **1**: 340–5

CALLAHAN CM, CITTUS RS, KATZ BP (1991) Oral corticosteroid therapy for patients with stable chronic obstructive pulmonary disease: a meta-analysis. *Annals of Internal Medicine* **114**: 216–23

ROBERTS CM, BUGLER JR, MELCHOR R et al. (1993) Value of pulse oximetry for long-term oxygen requirement. *European Respiratory Journal* **6**: 559–62

Assessment of disability

BORG G (1982) Psychophysical basis of perceived exertion. *Medicine and Science in Sports and Exercise* **14**: 377–81

MCGAVIN CR, ARTVINLI M, NAOE H (1978) Dyspnoea, disability and distance walked: a comparison of estimates of exercise performance in respiratory disease. *British Medical Journal* **2**: 241–3

NOSEDA A, CARPEIAUX JP, SCHMERBER J (1992) Dyspnoea assessed by visual analogue scale in patients with obstructive lung disease during progressive and high intensity exercise. *Thorax* **47**: 363–8

SINGH SJ, MORGAN MDL, SCOTT SC et al. (1992) The development of the shuttle walking test of disability in patients with chronic airways obstruction. *Thorax* **47**: 1019–24

WILLIAMS SJ, BURY MR (1989) Impairment, disability and handicap in chronic respiratory illness. *Social Science and Medicine* **29** (5): 609–16

Assessment of handicap

DUDLEY DL, GLASER EM, JORGENSON BN et al. (1980) Psychosocial concomitants to rehabilitation in chronic obstructive pulmonary disease. *Chest* **77** (3): 413–20

GUYATT GH, BERMAN LB, TOWNSEND M et al. (1987) A measure of quality of life for clinical trials in chronic lung disease. *Thorax* **42**: 773–8

HYLAND ME, BOTT J, SING S, KENYON CAP (1994) Domains, constructs and the development of the breathing problems questionnaire. *Quality of Life Research* **3**: 245–56

JONES PW, QUIRK FH, BAVEYSTOCK CM et al. (1992) A self-complete measure for chronic airflow limitation: the St George's questionnaire. *American Review of Respiratory Disease* **147**: 832–8

Addresses for questionnaires

Chronic Respiratory Disease Index Questionnaire
Gordon Guyatt
Department of Clinical Epidemiology and Biostatistics
McMaster University Medical Centre
1200 Main Street West
Hamilton, Ontario, CANADA L8N 3Z5

St George's Respiratory Questionnaire
Professor Paul Jones
Division of Physiological Medicine
St George's Hospital Medical School
Cranmer Terrace
London SW17 0RE

Breathing Problems Questionnaire
Professor Michael Hyland
Department of Psychology
University of Plymouth
Plymouth
Devon PL4 8AA

6 | Smoking cessation

Main points

1 Stopping smoking is the only intervention that significantly affects the natural history of COPD.

2 Advice from health professionals can be extremely effective in persuading patients to stop smoking.

3 The use of nicotine replacement therapy (NRT) can double long-term quit rates.

4 Matching patient to product may be helpful. Gum, inhalator, nasal spray or sublingual tablets may be most helpful for the heavily addicted smoker.

5 Support and follow-up of patients, particularly through the critical first two to three weeks, may also increase quit rates.

Stopping smoking is the single most important intervention in COPD and the only thing that significantly alters the natural history of the disease. It is of primary importance at every stage and must be encouraged actively and continuously. In mild COPD it may be the only treatment needed and may prevent the patient ever developing severe, disabling and life-threatening illness.

Unfortunately, persuading patients to stop smoking is often difficult, and failure can be demoralising and disheartening for patient and health professional alike. Most ex-smokers have made several serious attempts to stop before they eventually succeed. A 10% success rate is good!

Why do people smoke?

The reasons why patients start smoking and continue to smoke in the face of mounting evidence of its harmful effects are complex.

Currently 28% of adult males and 26% of adult females are smokers and 26% of the population are ex-smokers. Smoking rates are highest among lower socio-economic groups. Rising tobacco taxation and increasing evidence of the harmful effects of smoking have little effect on people in these groups. Perversely, those who can least afford it – the economically deprived – are those who tend to smoke, continue to smoke and smoke most!

Most smokers start in adolescence, when it may be seen as a 'rite of passage' to adulthood. There may be considerable and irresistible peer group pressure to smoke. Smoking may be one of those 'risk-taking' or rebellious behaviours that are a normal part of growing up. Unfortunately, a third of the adolescents who start will become life-long smokers, and 450 children start smoking every day. Health education messages about the long-term effects of smoking have little effect and the tobacco industry continues to spend large amounts of money persuading young smokers to begin. In the UK about 300 adults die of a smoking-related disease every day, so the tobacco industry needs to recruit new smokers to replace them!

Nicotine is highly addictive and smokers are adept at adjusting their smoking to satisfy their need for nicotine without taking in so much that they suffer side-effects. It is also a powerful neural stimulant, and enhances concentration and mental agility. Stimulation is followed by rebound depression and the addicted smoker then feels the need for another cigarette. Nicotine also reduces anxiety and can be used to 'calm the nerves'.

- The cigarette is a highly efficient nicotine-delivery system. Nicotine is absorbed very rapidly across the lungs and reaches the brain quicker than if it were injected intravenously.

- If the number of cigarettes smoked a day is reduced, the smoker will take longer and deeper puffs to get the same amount of nicotine.

- Reducing the number smoked or switching to a lower tar cigarette is seldom successful as a quitting strategy.

- Cigarette smokers who switch to cigars are likely to inhale the cigar smoke and get an even higher tar load into the lungs than with cigarettes.

Nicotine, although addictive, is a relatively harmless drug. It is the other constituents of tobacco that cause damage. Cigarette smoke contains upwards of 4,000 different chemicals, 600 of which are known carcinogens. Perrier water was withdrawn from sale when it was found to contain 4.7µg per litre of benzene, a known carcinogen. A single cigarette delivers 190µg of benzene!

Addiction to nicotine is only one reason why smokers find it hard to stop. Each cigarette is 'puffed' about 10–12 times, and 20 cigarettes a day is associated with 200–250 hand-to-mouth movements every day: 91,250 movements a year. A powerful habit! Smoking becomes associated with pleasurable everyday activities: having a cup of coffee, relaxing after a meal, watching the television etc. It may be associated with pleasurable memories and social activities. When smokers try to quit they not only have to cope with withdrawal of an addictive drug but also with the loss of an 'old friend' that might have been part of their lives for many years. Fear of failure may be another powerful reason why a smoker does not make any move to stop.

How can smokers stop smoking?

In order to stop, the smoker has to *want* to stop. This sounds painfully obvious but the path from 'contented' smoker to serious 'quitter' is tortuous and one where advice from you can have a considerable influence. Nearly 70% of smokers say they would like to stop, so constructive advice, support and encouragement might help them to move from a period of contemplation to doing something serious about quitting. Tagging the medical records and bringing up the subject of smoking in a non-threatening way at every attendance can be highly effective and may prompt a 'contented smoker' to contemplate stopping, or a smoker who is contemplating stopping to making a serious attempt to stop. Showing concern and offering support is perhaps most helpful. A censorious approach is likely to produce only resistance.

Smokers need to be informed of the risks they are taking in continuing to smoke, and that information needs to be relevant to them. In the case of COPD this should be relatively easy. Relating a COPD patient's own lung function to what it would be in a healthy non-smoker (see Figure 2.2) may provide a powerful incentive to take a serious step towards becoming an ex-smoker. A dramatic event (e.g. a myocardial infarction) that makes a patient anxious about their health is often a trigger to action. Unfortunately, slowly progressive breathlessness seldom produces the same trigger, but a recent unpleasant chest infection or exacerbation of COPD might. Targeting patients when they are most susceptible to advice may increase success rates.

Once a patient has decided to make a serious attempt to stop smoking, practical advice on how to cope and support through the first critical three months of stopping are most beneficial. 'Quit smoking' groups are available in some areas for people who feel they would benefit from a support group. (They are often organised by the Health Education Authority or a cancer prevention group.) Alternatively, follow-up appointments at the surgery or health centre at one week, three weeks, two months and three months after stopping to offer support and encouragement may be helpful. If your resources are strained, the most important period to concentrate on is the first month. It may take several serious attempts before a smoker makes the final transition to ex-smoker. In the event of relapse, it is important not to condemn but rather to support and encourage the patient to try to identify why they have failed, develop a strategy for avoiding failure in the future and to make another serious attempt. As Mark Twain famously remarked:

'Stopping smoking is easy. I've done it hundreds of times.'

Nicotine replacement therapy

For some smokers, withdrawal symptoms such as irritability, nervousness and cravings may cause relapse and unwillingness to make another attempt to quit. Nicotine replacement therapy (NRT) can be very effective; large, placebo-controlled trials have shown that it can double quit rates at one year. It is available in five forms:

- chewing gum,
- transdermal patch,
- inhaler,
- nasal spray,
- sublingual tablet.

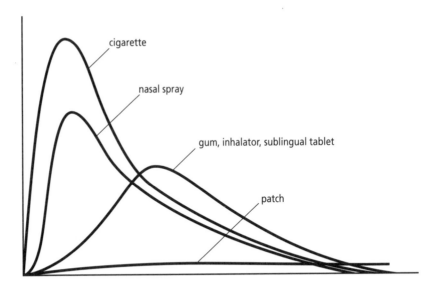

cigarette

nasal spray

gum, inhalator, sublingual tablet

patch

Figure 6.1 Blood nicotine levels with different types of nicotine replacement therapy

Figure 6.1 shows the different blood nicotine levels with the different types. Unfortunately, none of these products is available on NHS prescription. It is interesting that nicotine addiction is the only addiction for which you cannot be treated on the National Health Service! However, NRT is still cheaper than smoking and some areas have schemes that provide patients with their first week of NRT so that they can use the money saved in the first week to purchase the second and subsequent weeks of treatment.

Nicotine gum

This is the oldest form of NRT and is available over the counter in two strengths (2mg and 4mg) and a variety of flavours. The gum should be chewed until it starts to produce a flavour and then 'parked' between the cheek and the gum. If it is chewed continuously, it tastes unpleasant. When the desire to smoke is felt again, the gum is chewed and parked again. Each piece of gum lasts about 20 minutes and up to 16 pieces can be chewed in 24 hours. Nicotine is absorbed from the lining of the mouth, the buccal mucosa, and produces a peak in venous nicotine levels similar in shape but less than that achieved by smoking. It is suitable for the highly addicted smoker because it is used on demand.

Nasal spray

The peaks in nicotine level that can be achieved with a nasal spray are higher than can be obtained with the gum but still considerably lower than those achieved with cigarettes. The nicotine is absorbed from the nasal mucosa. It should not be sniffed up the nose but sprayed onto the mucosa when the desire to smoke is felt. Up to 64 'puffs' a day can be used. This form of NRT most closely resembles the effects of smoking and is most suitable for the very heavily addicted smoker. It is available only on private prescription.

Nicotine inhalator

The inhalator produces peaks in nicotine levels similar to those from nicotine gum. The inhalator contains a mentholated plug impregnated with nicotine, and is sucked when the desire to smoke is felt and until that desire goes away. Nicotine is absorbed from the buccal mucosa. Each plug lasts for about 20 minutes.

Nicotine patches

Transdermal patches are easy to use. They are of two types (16 hour or 24 hour), and come in several strengths. Patches do not produce peaks in nicotine levels to mimic the effect of smoking but, rather, provide a steady background level. The rationale behind the 24-hour patch is to prevent the strong urge to smoke that many smokers feel first thing in the morning, caused by an overnight fall in nicotine levels. They may, however, produce sleep disturbance or nightmares, and the adhesive in the patches can cause local skin irritation.

Sublingual tablets

Sublingual tablets are a recent addition to the range of NRT products available. When the desire to smoke is felt, a tablet is dissolved under the tongue. The peak in nicotine level obtained is similar to that achieved with gum or the inhalator, and, because they too are used on demand, sublingual tablets are suitable for heavily addicted smokers. Unlike the other forms of NRT, these tablets are licensed for use during pregnancy and for breast-feeding mothers.

The principle of NRT is to replace the nicotine a smoker takes in, although at considerably lower levels, thus reducing withdrawal symptoms and allowing the smoker to concentrate on changing the habits of smoking. When the habit is broken, the amount of nicotine can be reduced over a period and the NRT withdrawn. It is important that the smoker understands at the outset that it is not intended to replace cigarettes and will not be a substitute for will power. A considerable amount of nicotine will be given up from day one. In order for NRT to work, the smoker has to be motivated to stop! It is not suitable for the genuinely light or social smoker, because it may provide more nicotine than they are accustomed to and produce toxic side-effects.

To maximise success with NRT it may help if you match the smoker to the product and ensure that the smoker's expectations of the effects of NRT are realistic. Instruction in how to chew the gum or use the inhalator may prevent problems with incorrect use. Failure with NRT is often due to:

- stopping therapy too soon,

- not using high enough doses because of fears about side-effects,

- concurrent smoking – a potentially dangerous practice.

The list of possible side-effects on the side of a packet of NRT can be daunting. Fear of side-effects may also be used as an excuse not to attempt to stop smoking, and some smokers are concerned about becoming addicted to the NRT! This is in fact a rare occurrence, so you can reassure patients that this is unlikely, and, although undesirable, is still safer than continuing to smoke.

It is important that patients understand that the side-effects of NRT are the same as the side-effects of smoking but that the risks of using it are considerably less than those of continuing to smoke. Except for the sublingual tablets (see earlier), however, NRT should *not* be used by pregnant or breast-feeding women because of the lack of research into its teratogenicity. It is also advised that NRT not be used:

- within three months of a myocardial infarction,

- within three months of a cerebrovascular accident,

- by people with active peptic ulceration,

although for these patients the risks of continuing to smoke are probably considerably higher.

Transdermal patches should not be used by patients with extensive skin disease; the other types of NRT – chewing gum, nasal spray, inhalator or sublingual tablets – should be used instead.

Generally, NRT should be taken for 12 weeks with a two- to four-week period at the end of the course when the dose is reduced. The benefits of using NRT and stopping smoking massively outweigh the risks of continuing to smoke, and helping patients to come to grips with the reality of the risks may be helpful.

Helping patients to stop smoking can be the most rewarding and the most frustrating of tasks. However, it is the single most important thing you can do to improve the health of your patient. You must ask the smoker about their smoking habits and offer support and advice at every attendance. It is tempting sometimes not to bother to raise the subject because you know that you have discussed smoking cessation with that patient many times and your advice hasn't been heeded. But this may be the one time when you may make a difference! The following hints may be helpful.

Practical hints for health professionals

- Raise the subject of smoking cessation in a non-threatening way.

- Assess motivation to quit by asking questions such as 'How do you feel about stopping smoking?'

- Show concern and offer appropriate advice/leaflets to the 'contented' smoker.

- Discuss the benefits of nicotine replacement therapy. Help patients to select an appropriate form and teach them how to use it.

- Follow up smokers during their attempt to quit.

- If they don't succeed, encourage them to try again.

Practical hints for patients

1 *Set a 'quit' date.*
Stopping smoking is something you need to plan. It is seldom successful if it is undertaken on the spur of the moment, and gently cutting back is not effective. The best way to stop is just to stop.

Before quitting it may be helpful to keep a smoking diary so that danger times can be highlighted and strategies formulated for avoiding them.

Family and friends need to be informed so that they don't put temptation in your way. If possible, quit with a friend. Success rates are much higher when people have support and reinforcement available.

You may find the Quitline (Smokeline, in Scotland) helpful. Their telephone numbers are:

England: 0800 00 22 00
Northern Ireland: 02890 663 281
Scotland: 0800 84 84 84
Wales: 0345 697 500

2 *On 'quit day' get rid of all cigarettes, lighters and ash trays.*

3 *Cash, not ash.*
Put aside the money you would have spent on smoking and reward yourself after a week or a fortnight.

4 *Avoid replacing cigarettes with extra cups of coffee or tea.*
Caffeine levels will be increased when you stop smoking and unpleasant side-effects (e.g. headaches) may occur. It is better to drink plenty of water or fruit juice.

5 *Cravings are short lived.*
Try to avoid situations where you would normally smoke. For example, instead of sitting down with a cup of coffee after a meal, get up and do something different. It may be advisable to stay away from the pub or from friends who smoke for the critical first two or three weeks. Alcohol may also weaken your power to resist a cigarette. Work out ways to distract yourself when cravings occur, to occupy you until they pass.

6 *Keep a 'nibble box' of raw carrots, celery or some other non-fattening food.*
Weight gain is common (average weight gain is about 4 kilograms). Don't try to diet and quit smoking at the same time, but do try to avoid sucking sweets and eating fattening foods to overcome your craving for cigarettes. As you begin to feel fitter, try taking up some form of exercise. This will help to keep your weight down and improve your general fitness.

7 *Take it one day at a time.*
Tell yourself 'Today, I am not going to have a cigarette.'

8 *If you don't succeed this time – try again!*
Work out why you have failed and then try again. Learn from your mistakes.

Further reading

BRITISH THORACIC SOCIETY (1998) Smoking cessation guidelines and their cost effectiveness. *Thorax* **53** (Suppl 5): S1–38

NATIONAL ASTHMA AND RESPIRATORY TRAINING CENTRE (1999) *Simply Stop Smoking.* Direct Publishing Solutions, Cookham, Berks

PROCHASKA JO, DICLEMENTE CC (1986) Towards a comprehensive model of change. In: Miller WR, Heather N (eds) *Treating Addictive Behaviours: Process of change.* Plenum, New York

SILAGY C, MANT D, FOWLER G et al. (1994) Meta-analysis on efficacy of nicotine replacement therapies in smoking cessation. *Lancet* **343**: 139–42

7 Bronchodilators

Main points

1 Bronchodilators are the most important treatment for symptom relief in COPD.

2 They work by
   – decreasing bronchomotor tone,
   – decreasing lung hyperinflation,
   – decreasing the work of breathing.

3 They are most appropriately taken by inhalation, and have a rapid onset of action.

4 An inhaler device should be selected that the patient can use effectively.

5 The patient's inhaler technique should be checked at regular intervals.

6 Short-acting beta-agonists and anticholinergics are equally efficacious. Sometimes combined therapy may have an additive effect.

7 In severe COPD, bronchodilators should be taken regularly four-hourly. In some patients, higher doses may prove more beneficial.

8 Additional treatments to consider are:
   – long-acting beta-agonists,
   – theophyllines.

9 A small number of patients with severe COPD warrant a nebuliser trial.

Bronchodilators are the most important treatment in COPD. They form the cornerstone of therapy to improve symptoms and treat any reversible component of airflow obstruction.

There may seem to be a lack of logic in using lung function tests – FEV_1 or PEF – to predict symptomatic response to bronchodilators in COPD. By definition, a diagnosis of COPD implies that airflow obstruction is irreversible and so it is unlikely that the lung function will improve. However, a reversibility test to a single dose of bronchodilator that achieves a large improvement in lung function will help to identify patients with a significant asthmatic component to their disease.

Although reversibility testing is an essential part of the diagnostic process, a small or minimal change in lung function after a bronchodilator is not always a good predictor of the improvement that patients might experience. It is therefore most important to prescribe a trial of bronchodilators, either beta-agonist or anticholinergic inhalers, to be used regularly for three to four weeks. Such trials must be performed when the patient is stable.

The symptomatic response described by the patient will help to determine both the efficacy of treatment and which bronchodilator provides most improvement. Patients frequently notice:

- a decrease in shortness of breath,
- improved walking distance,
- an overall better quality of life.

Ways to assess these subjective improvements objectively are described in Chapter 5.

There is no single test of lung function that can accurately predict the degree of symptomatic improvement an individual can achieve with prolonged use of a bronchodilator. Perhaps the closest achievable for general practice is the forced vital capacity (FVC).

How do bronchodilators work?

Bronchodilators reverse the increased bronchomotor tone found in the airways of COPD patients by relaxing smooth muscle and thus reducing airway resistance. Several studies have shown improvements in vital capacity (VC) of 500ml or more, with a similar decrease in residual volume (RV) (see Chapter 4 and Figure 4.11).

Hyperinflation is reduced, and it is easier and more comfortable for the patient to breathe. Breathlessness and the effort of breathing are reduced, so patients can walk further.

Beta-agonists also promote an increase in mucociliary activity, but it is unlikely that this effect has any clinical importance. Theophyllines may, in addition, have a small effect on increasing respiratory muscle endurance, but again it is hard to assess whether this is of clinical significance.

Beta-agonists in high doses may also dilate pulmonary blood vessels. When ventilation of the lungs is impaired, as in acute exacerbations, this effect may cause a worsening of any ventilation/ perfusion mismatch and result in a small, transient fall in arterial oxygen levels.

Bronchodilator administration

As in asthma, the preferred way to use a bronchodilator is by inhalation. Although oral bronchodilators may be just as effective in providing symptom relief, they have the disadvantages of greater side-effects, potential drug interactions and a slower onset of action.

Metered dose inhalers (MDIs) are inexpensive and effective, working rapidly to provide symptom relief. Correct timing and co-ordination can make them difficult to use, and less than 50% of patients can inhale from them effectively. This is especially so in elderly patients, who may have other illnesses such as arthritis or dementia. With repeated tuition, or the addition of a large volume spacer or breath-activated MDI, the proportion of patients able to use MDIs effectively can be greatly increased.

Dry powder devices are simpler to use and equally effective but are more expensive. As in asthma, it is essential that patients are prescribed a device that they can use effectively and are assessed regularly for competence in its use. Patients should be involved in the initial choice of device.

Types of bronchodilator

Short-acting beta-agonists

These drugs have a rapid onset of action (usually within five minutes) and a duration of action of three to four hours, and are recommended for both regular treatment and 'as required' for relief of symptoms. They can also be used before exercise to increase exercise tolerance or to relieve breathlessness. More severe levels of airflow obstruction should be treated with beta-agonists four-hourly (or even more frequently in extreme cases). It is safe and sometimes more effective to give two or three times the standard dose to achieve a better therapeutic response.

The regular use of short-acting beta-agonists in severe COPD is thus quite different from the accepted policy for all but the most severe grades of asthma (steps 4 and 5 in the BTS *Guidelines for Asthma Management*), for which it is taught that they should be used only as required for symptom relief. Older patients may become less responsive to beta-agonists and may achieve a better improvement with an anticholinergic agent. As with any therapy, success or failure of a given agent should be assessed both objectively, with tests of lung function, and subjectively, from the point of view of the patient's perceived response over a month of treatment. Alternatives or additions may then need to be explored.

Anticholinergic agents

Anticholinergics have a slower onset of action (15–30 minutes) than short-acting beta-agonists (5 minutes) but the results of most comparative studies suggest that they are equally effective in achieving symptom relief. Indeed, in some they have produced a greater response and a longer duration of bronchodilation. The responses of individual patients to both anticholinergic and short-acting beta-agonist bronchodilators should therefore be assessed.

Combined therapy

The use of short-acting beta-agonist with an anticholinergic may have an additive effect in some patients. Combined therapy may produce greater improvements in exercise tolerance and a greater degree of bronchodilation than either drug used separately.

If patients' symptoms improve with a combination of salbutamol and ipratropium, there is a clinical advantage in giving the drugs in a combined inhaler. Patients may find this more convenient and compliance may be enhanced.

Long-acting beta-agonists

Inhaled Long-acting beta-agonists have a duration of action of 12 hours. When taken twice daily they have produced good improvements in symptoms and peak flow in asthmatics who are already taking moderate doses of inhaled steroids. Recent studies with salmeterol in COPD have shown improvements in breathlessness, sleep quality and lung function, as well as in scores of overall quality of life. A recent Cochrane review of long-acting beta-agonists in COPD comments that, although there are only small increases in FEV_1, some patients show good improvements in breathlessness and quality of life. FEV_1 change does not correlate well with clinical improvements, so the study recommends that the agents be used in patients who report a definite improvement while on therapy.

Comparative studies with both short-acting beta-agonists and anticholinergics have reported similar improvements in lung function, but the duration of action of salmeterol is considerably longer; a twice-daily regimen might enhance compliance in some patients. More studies are required for a fuller appraisal, but the long-acting inhaled beta-agonists are likely to be of benefit in COPD if the individual patient's symptoms improve.

Oral The use of oral long-acting beta-agonists in COPD also needs further study, but they may occasionally be justified for a patient with severe COPD who has difficulty using any form of inhaled therapy. If they are used, care must be taken to ensure that there is no significant side-effect such as tremor, tachycardia or hypokalaemia and that coexisting angina is not being made worse.

Theophyllines

Theophyllines produce only small amounts of bronchodilation in COPD and tend to be most effective in the higher parts of the narrow therapeutic range (i.e. blood levels of 10–20mg/litre). They can increase exercise tolerance, and some patients report a good improvement in symptoms. Other effects reported in research studies – such as an anti-inflammatory action, improvements in respiratory muscle strength and improvements in right ventricular performance – are difficult to evaluate clinically. If theophyllines are used, it is preferable to give them in a slow-release form, and to monitor serum theophylline levels regularly.

Side-effects such as nausea, headache and palpitations are common and there are also interactions with anti-epileptic drugs, diltiazem, verapamil, frusemide, erythromycin, ciprofloxacin and cimetidine, to name but a few. Blood levels are also influenced by smoking, viral infections, influenza vaccination and impaired renal and hepatic function. In elderly patients with multiple co-pathologies it can be extremely difficult to achieve an effective and stable blood level of theophylline. The risk/benefit ratio must therefore be considered carefully.

Nebulised bronchodilators

A small number of patients with severe COPD do not show any symptomatic improvement with inhaled bronchodilators, even with multiple doses taken through a large volume spacer. Sometimes benefit can be achieved only by using higher doses via a nebuliser. Nebulised bronchodilators are generally more expensive. They are also less convenient to administer because they take longer and a power source is usually required, although some nebuliser/compressor systems have rechargeable battery packs or run off a car cigarette lighter thus allowing the patient greater flexibility and mobility.

Nebuliser therapy

Nebulisers are devices that convert a drug solution into a continuous fine aerosol of sufficiently small particle size to penetrate to all levels of the airways. Drug inhalation is achieved by the patient breathing normally (tidal breathing) through the nebuliser over a five to ten minute period. The advantage of a nebuliser is that it can deliver a large dose of drug simply, particularly to patients who are too breathless or unwell to use a normal inhaler device effectively, or who have benefited clinically from higher doses.

The most commonly used varieties of nebuliser are:

- the standard jet nebuliser,
- the more advanced and efficient breath-assisted nebulisers, such as the Ventstream,
- the ultrasonic nebuliser.

The first two of these need to be driven by a compressor delivering flow rates of 6–8 litres per minute. Ultrasonic nebulisers contain a piezo crystal that vibrates at high speed, agitating the nebuliser solution so that it breaks up into particles small enough to be inhaled. They are smaller, quicker and quieter than the more commonly used jet nebuliser/compressor systems but they are also more expensive. A recent innovation, adaptive aerosol delivery, delivers the drug during inhalation only, thus eliminating waste of drug during exhalation, and can be programmed to deliver a precise dose. It costs more than both the standard nebuliser/compressor system and the ultrasonic nebuliser. If delivery of a precise amount of drug is not of paramount importance, it may not be a cost-effective option.

A mouthpiece is usually preferred to a facemask to deliver the nebulised mist. This is because there is a small risk of precipitating glaucoma when ipratropium or a combination of ipratropium and salbutamol is used via a facemask.

If a nebuliser/compressor system is supplied for long-term use at home, patients and their carers need to be given written instructions about cleaning and maintaining the equipment. Nebuliser chamber and mouthpiece or facemask need to be washed in warm soapy water and dried thoroughly after each use. The small jet holes can be dried by attaching the nebuliser to the compressor and running the compressor for about ten seconds to remove any residual fluid. Standard disposable nebuliser chambers will last a single patient for three months of regular use before they become inefficient and need to be replaced. Tubing should not be washed inside because it is impossible to dry it effectively. Nebuliser equipment that is stored damp may constitute an infection risk.

Compressors need to be serviced regularly, according to manufacturer's instructions. An annual electrical safety check is the legal responsibility of whoever supplies the compressor. When compressor systems are supplied by a pharmaceutical company on a named patient basis, it is the responsibility of the doctor who recommended it to ensure that it is electrically safe.

In the surgery, standard nebulisers, tubing and masks are for single use only and should then be discarded. It is not possible to sterilise them effectively and there is thus a risk of passing infection from one patient to another. For medico-legal purposes, it is advisable to adhere to the single-use policy. 'Durable' nebulisers are made by some manufacturers; these can be sterilised effectively in an autoclave and used for a year. They may be more cost-effective than single-use disposable nebulisers. Maintenance of equipment should follow the manufacturer's recommendations.

Nebuliser trials

The BTS *Nebuliser Guidelines* require patients to attempt high-dose bronchodilator therapy with up to six to eight puffs four-hourly through a large volume spacer before undertaking a formal nebuliser trial. Multiple 'puffs' of bronchodilator are given through a spacer, with the patient inhaling each puff separately. Assessment for the appropriate use of a nebuliser should follow BTS Guidelines for nebuliser therapy and be carried out by a hospital specialist or a GP with experience of nebuliser trials. Nebulised beta-agonists and anticholinergics should be tried alone and then in combination in order to determine which therapy produces the best effect.

To perform a nebuliser trial the patient should be clinically stable. A suggested protocol is:

- Week 1: large volume spacer and high-dose bronchodilator

- Week 2: nebulised short-acting beta-agonist (e.g. salbutamol 2.5–5mg or terbutaline 5–10mg four times a day)

- Week 3: nebulised anticholinergic (e.g. ipratropium bromide 250–500µg four times a day)

- Week 4: nebulised combined short-acting beta-agonist and anticholinergic (e.g. salbutamol 5mg + ipratropium 500µg four times a day)

Patients should perform serial peak flow tests during the trial. A positive response is either an increase in lung function (improvement of 15% in peak flow during the trial) or a definite improvement in symptoms on active treatment. If a nebuliser is helpful, a nebuliser/compressor unit should be provided by the local chest clinic, who will:

- educate the patient and their carer(s) in its use,

- provide regular maintenance of the unit,

- supply disposables such as the nebuliser chamber, and

- provide emergency back-up in the event of breakdown.

Unfortunately, the provision of properly organised, hospital-based nebuliser services is patchy at best. In many areas of the UK, patients (or their GPs) are expected to purchase and maintain nebulisers for long-term use. This situation is far from satisfactory.

Bronchodilator therapy can improve a COPD patient's symptoms without necessarily producing significant changes in lung function. All patients should undergo therapeutic trials with different bronchodilators and different combinations of bronchodilators at different doses in order to determine which drug (or drugs) produces the best therapeutic response. A general guide to the use of bronchodilators with increasingly severe disease is given in Table 7.1.

Table 7.1 Bronchodilator use with increasing severity of COPD

Mild	No treatment needed
(FEV$_1$ 60–80%)	For symptom relief, beta-agonist or anticholinergic as required
Moderate	Beta-agonist or anticholinergic 1–4 times daily,
(FEV$_1$ 40–59%)	as symptoms dictate
	Usually only one inhaler is needed
Severe	Regular beta-agonists or anticholinergics or
(FEV$_1$ below 40%)	combined beta-agonists and anticholinergics
	Some patients may benefit from higher doses of beta-agonists or anticholinergics
	Consider the addition of long-acting beta-agonists or theophyllines
	Consider a nebuliser trial

Further reading

General

British Thoracic Society (1997) BTS Guidelines for the management of chronic obstructive pulmonary disease. *Thorax* **52** (Suppl 5): S1–28

British Thoracic Society (1997) Current best practice for nebuliser treatment. *Thorax* **52** (Suppl 2): S1–106

Nisar M, Walshaw M, Earis JE, Pearson M, Calverley PMA (1990) Assessment of reversibility of airway obstruction in patients with chronic obstructive airways disease. *Thorax* **45**: 190–4.

Short-acting beta-agonists

BELLAMY D, HUTCHISON DCS (1981) The effects of salbutamol aerosol on the lung function of patients with emphysema. *British Journal of Diseases of the Chest* **75**: 190–5

VAN SCHAYCK CP, DOMPELING E, VAN HERWAARDEN CLA, FOLGERING H, VERBEEK AL, VAN DER HOOGEN HJ (1991) Bronchodilator treatment in moderate asthma or chronic bronchitis; continuous or on demand. A randomised controlled study. *British Medical Journal* **303**: 1426–31

Anticholinergics

ANTHONISEN NR, CONNETT JE, KILEY JP et al. (1994) Effects of smoking intervention and the use of an inhaled anticholinergic bronchodilator on the rate of decline of FEV_1. *Journal of the American Medical Association* **272**: 1497–505

BRAUN SR, MCKENZIE WN, COPELAND C, KNIGHT I, ELLERSIECK M (1989) A comparison of the effect of ipratropium and albuterol in the treatment of chronic airways disease. *Archives of Internal Medicine* **149**: 544–7

COMBIVENT INHALATION AEROSOL STUDY (1994) Combination of ipratropium and albuterol is more effective than either agent alone. *Chest* **105**: 1411–19

Long-acting beta-agonists

BOYD G, MORICE AH, POUNDSFORD JC, SIEBERT M, PESLIS N, CRAWFORD C (1997) An evaluation of salmeterol in the treatment of chronic obstructive airways disease. *European Respiratory Journal* **10**: 815–21

JONES PW, BOSH TK (1997) Quality of life changes in COPD patients treated with salmeterol. *American Journal of Respiratory and Critical Care Medicine* **155**: 1283–9

Theophyllines

MCKAY SE, HOWIE CA, THOMSON AH, WHITING B, ADDIS GJ (1993) Value of theophylline treatment in patients handicapped by chronic obstructive pulmonary disease. *Thorax* **48**: 227–32

Corticosteroid therapy

Main points

1 Inflammatory changes exist in the airways of patients with COPD, with increases in neutrophils, T-lymphocytes and macrophages. These inflammatory changes are different from those in asthma.

2 The effect of steroids has not been well studied pathologically, and the clinical response is often limited or negligible.

3 The BTS Guidelines suggest that only 10–20% of patients tested respond positively to oral prednisolone 30mg a day for two weeks. Those who do respond should be treated with long-term inhaled steroids. Steroid reversibility testing is a problematic issue in terms of its ability to determine treatment outcomes in COPD, but it does help to identify potential asthmatics. (Since the BTS Guidelines were written in 1995 there have been major new studies relating to inhaled steroid therapy. Points 4–8 relate to these studies.)

4 The short-term effects (up to six months) may be different from the long-term effects of corticosteroid treatment.

5 For a person to be classed as having a positive response to corticosteroids there should be an improvement in symptoms, fewer exacerbations and improved quality of life in the short term.

6 The Isolde study indicates that high-dose inhaled steroids improve clinical symptoms over three years, but the effect on the decline in lung function is much less impressive. The Euroscop and Copenhagen long-term studies failed to show a clinically meaningful response or a significant improvement in lung function.

7 A recently published meta-analysis of the effect of inhaled corticosteroids on lung function over two years suggests a small improvement in the treated group compared with those given a placebo, but only at high dosage. This might help to explain the differences in response between the large studies (Euroscop and Isolde), and perhaps indicates that high doses will be required to effect a worthwhile result. This dose-related effect was noted in early studies using oral steroids.

8 When assessing the efficacy of corticosteroids, changes in symptoms and health status should be considered as well as the FEV_1.

9 These important inhaled corticosteroid studies are first summarised below, and then followed by a more detailed appraisal.

In asthma, there is abundant evidence that the chronic inflammatory changes in the mucosa of the airways can be made histologically normal with both oral and inhaled corticosteroids. However, although the symptoms of most patients with COPD will improve with bronchodilator therapy, their response to corticosteroids is far less clear-cut. Although chronic inflammation is present in the small airways, there is little histological evidence of the effects that steroids may have on it. The situation is complicated because COPD is a spectrum of diseases ranging from the more obvious inflammation of chronic bronchitis to the destructive changes in the alveoli and supportive tissues in emphysema. Responses to steroid treatment will vary accordingly.

The rationale for using corticosteroids

The chronic inflammatory changes in the small airways of patients with COPD include increases both in the number of neutrophils and lymphocytes and in the number and activity of alveolar macrophages. The neutrophil is thought to be the most important cell in the pathogenesis of lung damage. Smokers with normal lung function often have increased neutrophils and macrophages.

The inflammation in asthma is characterised by thickening of the basement membrane as well as increased eosinophils and mast cells. These changes are not found in COPD, which suggests a different type of inflammatory process.

The BTS Guidelines advice on inhaled steroids in COPD

The BTS *COPD Guidelines* suggest that all patients with moderate or severe COPD (FEV_1 below 60% predicted) should have a formal steroid reversibility test. Prednisolone 30mg per day is given for two weeks, and the patient's lung function is measured both at the start and at the completion of the test period. Increases of FEV_1 of more than 200ml and 15% over baseline represent a positive response. Another way to perform the steroid reversibility test is to give beclomethasone (or an equivalent steroid) 500µg twice daily for six weeks. Patients who respond positively should be treated for the rest of their lives with:

- beclomethasone 1000µg per day,
- budesonide 800µg per day, or
- fluticasone 500µg per day.

There is little evidence that two weeks of prednisolone is an adequate period for a steroid trial. Neither is there any clear evidence-based guidance as to whether patients already on inhaled steroids should undergo a steroid challenge test before or after tailing of their inhaled steroid.

Only 10–20% of patients respond positively, and the BTS Guidelines suggest that there are no grounds for starting inhaled steroids with the other 80–90%. There may be no justification for continuing inhaled steroids in a patient who was incorrectly diagnosed as having asthma but in fact has COPD. The inhaled steroid should be reduced gradually over at least one to two months, monitoring closely the patient's clinical response and lung function. If the patient's condition deteriorates, the inhaled steroid should be reinstated.

New clinical information on inhaled steroids

Since the publication of the BTS Guidelines a number of important studies on the action of and response to inhaled steroids in COPD have been either published or presented at major meetings. While providing more information, the findings conflict with the views given in the BTS Guidelines. When evaluating the results of trials and studies, therefore, it is important to look at the outcomes being measured. For example:

- An improvement in symptoms and in quality of life.

- A reduction in the number of exacerbations.

- An improvement in lung function in the short term (six months).

- Slowing the rate of decline of lung function in the longer term (usually over three years).

Summary of the messages from the new studies

- In the short term, there are clinically significant improvements in lung function and symptoms, with fewer acute exacerbations. The results from the Isolde study indicate that these improvements are maintained for three years.

- There is relatively little or no change in the rate of decline of lung function (FEV_1) over three years with various inhaled steroids in moderate to high dosage (Euroscop, Isolde, Copenhagen Lung Study and the 1999 meta-analysis).

- The decline in quality of life is significantly slowed over a three-year period by high-dose fluticasone (Isolde).

- The more positive clinical responses tend to occur only with higher dose inhaled steroids (meta-analysis, Isolde).

What are the implications for primary care?

The results of the studies suggest that inhaled steroids have minimal effect on the long-term decline of lung function, and that the very small changes reported from some studies may or may not be clinically beneficial. However, there is growing evidence indicating worthwhile improvement in health status and symptoms and a reduction in the number of exacerbations. This is of considerable interest to patients.

As often happens with major studies that set out to answer important clinical questions, the results sometimes raise further issues and questions about how to treat patients. Some of the questions include:

- Isolde used high-dose fluticasone – would a smaller dose have had the same effect?

- Do all inhaled steroids produce the same benefit?

- At what stage should patients be given inhaled steroids – presumably when they have symptoms?

- What are the cost/benefits of long-term inhaled steroids?

- Is there a way to identify which patients are more likely to respond to treatment and which are not?

- If all symptomatic patients are to be treated with inhaled steroids, is it necessary to perform a steroid reversibility test?

The answers to these and other questions are far from clear. The sensible approach at present is to follow the advice given in the current BTS Guidelines and wait for the new evidence-based update due in 2001.

Is there a role for long-term oral steroids?

Most GP practices have patients with severe COPD who take oral steroids, usually for acute exacerbations. However, because of the potential side-effects, the BTS Guidelines do not recommend the regular use of oral steroids. When the steroids are gradually stopped, the patient may deteriorate rapidly, with worsening dyspnoea, cough or wheeze. So a further course of steroids is given. If the symptoms become worse as the steroids are again reduced, this usually indicates the need for ongoing oral steroid therapy. Such circumstances usually guide the decision to continue oral steroids unless or until their side-effects outweigh the benefits. Each patient needs to be counselled about the advantages and disadvantages of steroid therapy in relation to the severity of their disease, likely benefits and the side-effects, and should be involved in the decision whether to continue. My (DB) view is that oral steroids should be continued long term if:

■ they seem to have a definite clinical benefit,

■ the patient's quality of life is improved,

■ the patient has a life expectancy of two years or less.

The likelihood of serious side-effects is fairly small when a low dosage is used, preferably 10mg of prednisolone or less per day. For higher doses it may be necessary to consider using biphosphonates to prevent accelerated osteoporosis.

Steroids for acute exacerbations

It is common practice in primary and secondary care to treat exacerbations of COPD with courses of prednisolone, particularly when the symptoms are increasing breathlessness, wheeze and chest tightness. Symptoms usually return to baseline levels over one to three weeks and, as with acute asthma, the steroid treatment may need to be continued for up to 21 days.

Do corticosteroids have particular side-effects in COPD?

The side-effects of inhaled and systemic steroids are summarised in Table 8.1. Four factors are relevant to the use of corticosteroids in COPD:

■ Patients are generally older.

■ Most patients have a significant smoking history.

■ Those with severe COPD have a limited life expectancy.

■ Most receive a relatively small dose of corticosteroid.

Table 8.1 Side-effects of corticosteroids

Inhaled	Systemic
Oral candidiasis	Suppressed hypothalamic–pituitary–adrenal function
Dysphonia	Osteoporosis
Bruising	Hypertension
?Cataracts	Cataracts
	Weight gain
	Dyspepsia
	Cushingoid appearance
	Mood change
	Peripheral oedema
	Risk of diabetes
	Myopathy

Inhaled steroids seem to cause only minor side-effects, apart from mild oral and laryngeal problems and an increased risk of bruising. Oral steroids cause suppression of pituitary–adrenal function but this side-effect is probably of little clinical importance. Perhaps the main concern in severe COPD is the potential added effect on bone thinning from smoking and inactivity. Unfortunately, there have not yet been any controlled studies that specifically addressed these questions.

Synopsis of important clinical trials of inhaled steroids in COPD

Short-term trials

The study of **Dompeling et al.** (1992) examined a mixed group of asthma and COPD patients with known more rapid decline in lung function than usual. All patients were treated for a year with beclomethasone 800µg daily together with either salbutamol or ipratropium. In the patients with COPD there was a significant improvement in the rate of decline of FEV_1 in the first six months of treatment, but from months 7 to 12 the rate of decline returned to pre-steroid treatment levels. There was no change in the number of exacerbations but a small improvement in the symptoms of cough, sputum and dyspnoea. This study thus suggests small improvements in symptoms and slowed rate of decline in FEV_1 in the first six months that subsequently revert to pre-steroid treatment levels.

The two-year study by **Renkema et al.** (1996) examined 58 non-allergic patients with COPD. They were given:

- budesonide 1600µg per day, or
- budesonide 1600µg per day plus oral prednisolone 5mg per day, or
- a placebo.

As with the Dompeling study, there was a small but significant improvement in symptoms but no change in the number of exacerbations. The rate of decline of FEV_1 was:

- budesonide only: 30ml per year,
- budesonide plus prednisolone: 40ml per year,
- placebo: 60ml per year.

Because of a wide scatter of results, none of the differences reached statistical significance. The authors concluded that, over all, the benefits of the steroids were small but that some patients might achieve worthwhile responses. More studies are required to determine which COPD patients should receive inhaled steroids.

A recent multi-centre study by **Paggiaro et al.** (1998) compared fluticasone 1000µg per day with a placebo in 281 patients over a six-month period. These patients generally had more severe COPD than those in the studies described above. Outcome measures were symptom scores, exacerbations and lung function. Compared with the placebo group, the active treatment group had:

- fewer exacerbations ($p < 0.001$),
- improved symptom scores,
- a greater walking distance,
- improved peak flow and FEV_1.

This study also indicates a short-term improvement with inhaled corticosteroids, but the dose of fluticasone was high and probably more than would customarily be used in general practice. We do not know whether this response would have continued if the study had been extended for a further year.

In complete contrast, a recent study from Canada by **Bourbeau et al.** (1998) has shown no response to budesonide 1600µg per day over six months. This was also a placebo-controlled trial but the patients included had severe, advanced COPD. Initially, all patients received prednisolone 40mg per day for two weeks, and only those who were deemed steroid non-responders entered the double-blind phase of the study. Only 13.5% of the original 140 patients were designated steroid responders. There were no differences in FEV_1, symptom scores or quality of life scores between the treatment and the placebo groups.

These studies help to demonstrate the difficulty in interpreting the efficacy of inhaled steroids and the importance of knowing the selection criteria for the patients studied. The Canadian study lends weight to the conclusions in the BTS *COPD Guidelines* – that only patients who respond positively to a formal prednisolone trial should be given inhaled steroids long term. The other studies discussed did not differentiate between prednisolone responders and non-responders. The Dompeling study had patients with milder COPD; moreover, some of them were atopic and thus more likely to respond to the steroid. Over all, though, there seems to be a favourable short-term effect on symptoms in the first six months. The longer term changes in the rate of decline of lung function are, however, minimal.

Longer term studies

Two early studies by **Postma** (1985, 1988) reviewed retrospectively a group of patients with severe COPD for between 2 and 20 years. The patients who had regularly been taking oral prednisolone 10mg or more per day had a slower decline in FEV_1. If, however, the dose of prednisolone was reduced to less than 10mg per day, the FEV_1 tended to fall more rapidly. It is therefore important to balance the clinical benefits with the likely increasing number of side-effects from oral steroid therapy. At present, only patients with severe COPD would be considered for long-term oral steroids.

Multi-centre studies

Three major multi-centre studies have recently been completed. Each addressed the longer term effect of inhaled steroids on the decline of lung function compared with a control group.

Euroscop (European Respiratory Society, 1998) was a large European placebo-controlled study examining the effect of budesonide 800μg per day on the rate of decline of lung function over a three-year period. Entry criteria to the study included being a current smoker with a FEV_1/FVC ratio less than 70% and less than 10% reversibility following a course of prednisolone. Initially, 2147 people were recruited; those who stopped smoking or were non-compliant during the run-in period were dropped from the study, leaving 1277 participants. They had a mean age of 52 years and a mean FEV_1% predicted of 77% – mild COPD. The primary outcome variable was post-bronchodilator FEV_1.

The results revealed relatively small differences between the two groups. The overall three-year decline in FEV_1 was 140ml in the budesonide group and 180ml in the placebo group.

As in other studies, there was an initial improvement over the first six months with the inhaled steroid, followed by a similar decline from 9 to 36 months. Subgroup analysis revealed that:

- women did better than men,

- heavier smokers declined more rapidly,

- atopy had no significant role.

The overall conclusion was that the inhaled steroid had a limited long-term benefit on the rate of decline in lung function.

Isolde (European Respiratory Society, 1998) This British study compared fluticasone 500μg twice daily (via MDI and large volume spacer) with a placebo in moderate to severe COPD over a three-year period. The participants were older (mean age 64) and heavy smokers (44 pack-years). Outcome measures were:

- post-bronchodilator FEV_1,

- frequency of exacerbations,

- withdrawal from the study for respiratory reasons,

- health status scores.

After a two-month run-in period to obtain baseline levels, participants were given an oral prednisolone challenge and then randomised to fluticasone (376 patients, of whom 219 completed) or placebo (375 patients, of whom 182 completed). The mean FEV_1% predicted was 50% with steroid reversibility of 6%.

The difference in the *total rate of decline of FEV$_1$* over the three years was greater than in the Euroscop study, with values of 133ml for the fluticasone group and 197ml for the placebo group ($p =$ 0.0003). In the fluticasone group, the improvement peaked at six to nine months. Thereafter the annual decline in FEV$_1$ was fairly similar at 50ml for fluticasone and 59ml for placebo.

Exacerbation rates were lower on fluticasone (0.99 per year vs 1.33 on placebo) and there were more *withdrawals for respiratory causes* in the placebo group.

Health status was assessed using the St George's Questionnaire, which correlates well with respiratory symptoms but less well with FEV$_1$. A significant clinical change on this scale corresponds to four 'units'. Participants receiving fluticasone had a significantly slower rate of decline in health status than did those on placebo. A deterioration of four units occurred every 11 months in the placebo group, against 21 months in the fluticasone group. Thus, in this study of patients with moderate to severe COPD, high-dose fluticasone resulted in fewer exacerbations, improved symptoms and a better quality of life throughout the period of the study. The effect on the rate of decline in lung function was small, particularly over the last two years of the study.

Copenhagen Lung Study (Vestbo et al., 1999) This three-year Danish study compared budesonide 800µg per day (via turbohaler) with a placebo. The patients recruited for it had very mild impairment of lung function (FEV$_1$% predicted 86%); indeed, many of them would not match the BTS Guidelines definition of COPD. However, they were all heavy smokers. Out of 416 patients, 395 had no response to an initial trial with prednisolone.

At the end of the study, the decline in FEV$_1$ was almost identical: 46ml per year for the group receiving budesonide and 49ml per year for the placebo group – indicating no significant clinical benefit from budesonide over three years. However, the selection of steroid non-responders and an initial six months of high-dose budesonide would minimise any effect.

Inhaled corticosteroid meta-analysis (Van Grunsven et al. 1999) This combined Dutch–French meta-analysis looked at the effects of inhaled steroids in placebo-controlled trials over a two-year period. It identified three studies – two published and one in abstract form – and reanalysed the original data to conform to a more uniform format. Patients were included only if they had definite COPD.

The results show a small improvement of FEV_1 of 34ml per year in favour of the group receiving inhaled steroids. There was no difference in exacerbation rates in the two groups. The patients in the studies using high-dose steroids (beclomethasone 1500µg per day) did better than those on lower doses (budesonide 800µg per day), in whom there was little effect.

The authors of the paper conclude that this is the first published study to show a preservation of FEV_1 during two years of treatment, but only with high doses of inhaled steroid. This important study adds weight to the provisional early reports from the Isolde study that high-dose inhaled steroids seem to have a beneficial effect on long-term COPD; lower doses apparently do not.

Further reading

General

BRITISH THORACIC SOCIETY (1997) BTS Guidelines for the management of chronic obstructive pulmonary disease. *Thorax* **52** (Suppl 5): S1–28

JARAD NA, WEDZICHA JA, BURGE PS et al. (1999) An observational study of inhaled corticosteroid withdrawal in stable chronic obstructive pulmonary disease. *Respiratory Medicine* **93**: 161–6

MCEVOY CE, NIEWOEHNER DE (1997) Adverse effects of corticosteroid therapy for COPD – a critical review. *Chest* **111**: 732–43

THOMPSON WH, NIELSON CP, CARVALHO P et al. (1996) Controlled trial of oral prednisolone in outpatients with acute COPD exacerbation. *American Journal of Respiratory and Critical Care Medicine* **154**: 407–12

Short-term trials

BOURBEAU J, ROULEAU MY, BOUCHER S (1998) Randomised controlled trial of inhaled corticosteroids in patients with COPD. *Thorax* **53**: 447–82

DOMPELING E, VAN SCHAYK CP, MOLEMA J et al. (1992) Inhaled beclomethasone improves the course of asthma and COPD. *European Respiratory Journal* **5**: 945–52

PAGGIARO PL, DAHLE R, BAKRAN I et al. (1998) Multicentre randomised placebo controlled trial of inhaled fluticasone in patients with COPD. *Lancet* **351**: 773–9

RENKEMA TEJ, SCHOUTEN MS, KOETER GH, POSTMA DS (1996) Effects of long term treatment with corticosteroids in COPD. *Chest* **109**: 1156–62

Long-term trials

POSTMA DS, STEENHUIS EJ, VANDERWEELE LT et al. (1985) Severe chronic airflow obstruction: can corticosteroids slow down progression? *European Journal of Respiratory Disease* **67**: 56–64

POSTMA DS, PETERS I, STEENHUIS EJ et al. (1988) Moderately severe chronic airflow obstruction: can corticosteroids slow down progression? *European Respiratory Journal* **1**: 22–6

VAN GRUNSVEN PM, VAN SCHAYCK CP, DERENNE JP et al. (1999) Long term effects of inhaled corticosteroids in chronic obstructive pulmonary disease: a meta-analysis. *Thorax* **54**: 7–14

VESTBO J, SORENSEN T, LANGE P et al. (1999) Long-term effects of inhaled budesonide in mild and moderate chronic obstructive pulmonary disease: a randomised controlled trial. *Lancet* **353**: 1819–23

9 Pulmonary rehabilitation

Main points

1 Pulmonary rehabilitation improves exercise tolerance, dyspnoea and health status in people with COPD and may reduce their need for health care.

2 The cornerstone of rehabilitation is individually prescribed exercise endurance training.

3 Exercise for specific muscle groups can improve functional ability and may be particularly useful for patients with very severe disease.

4 Education about the disease and its management, nutrition, relaxation and coping strategies, and the management of exacerbations should also be included.

5 The patient's carer should be actively encouraged to be involved in the rehabilitation programme.

6 Support and encouragement to continue with lifestyle changes at the end of the programme are helpful.

7 *All patients benefit from keeping active.*

Historically, the management of COPD has focused on strategies either to prevent deterioration (stopping smoking) or to improve lung function (using bronchodilators and corticosteroids). Treatment that aimed to improve quality of life or health status and functional ability received little attention.

Now, however, there is increasing recognition that interventions can be made to improve patients' health status and to improve their ability to live with their condition. The nature of COPD – *fixed or partially fixed airflow obstruction* – means that improvement in lung function (impairment) can be at best modest, whereas improvement in patients' functional performance and health status (disability and handicap) can be considerable. Pulmonary rehabilitation focuses on these areas.

Evidence for the effectiveness of rehabilitation in COPD

A dictionary definition of rehabilitation is:

> 'to restore to good condition; to make fit after disablement or illness'.

Rehabilitation aims to restore the individual to the best physical, mental and emotional state possible. The ethos of rehabilitation has been embraced enthusiastically in the fields of cardiology, orthopaedics and neurology. In the UK, however, it has been adopted only slowly in respiratory medicine even though published guidelines from the European Respiratory Society, the American Thoracic Society and the British Thoracic Society state that rehabilitation is an important part of COPD management.

Whether pulmonary rehabilitation has an effect on mortality from COPD is controversial. It seems that the most important factor in determining survival is the post-bronchodilator FEV_1. However, maximal exercise capacity is also a factor in determining the prognosis in a patient with COPD, and pulmonary rehabilitation that improves maximal exercise capacity may also have a beneficial effect on mortality. It must be borne in mind, though, that extending the life of a COPD patient is not the prime aim of rehabilitation. Rather, it is to improve the quality and reduce the dependence of their remaining years.

There is plenty of evidence that pulmonary rehabilitation is effective in reducing breathlessness and improving exercise tolerance. Controlled studies have revealed that the sensation of dyspnoea is reduced and exercise capacity is increased after exercise training, and health-related quality of life scores also improve following rehabilitation programmes.

Evidence that pulmonary rehabilitation reduces the need for health care has come largely from the USA. There, programmes are eligible for reimbursement by insurers because they have been found to substantially reduce both hospital admission rates and inpatient stays. There has been little motivation to reduce the cost of emergency admissions for COPD in the UK but, with recent NHS reforms, this situation is likely to change. Obviously, the financial saving to the health service depends on the cost of the rehabilitation programme, but they are generally 'low tech' and cheap compared with the cost of admitting a patient to hospital because of an exacerbation of COPD.

Why rehabilitation programmes are needed

Breathlessness on exertion and the fear, anxiety and panic it engenders often lead a person with COPD to avoid activity. Attacks of breathlessness or coughing that occur outside the home may cause particular anxiety and embarrassment. Exercise avoidance results in

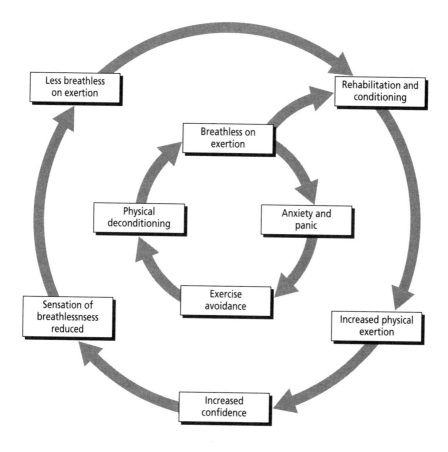

Figure 9.1 The effects of activity or inactivity on exercise tolerance.
(Reproduced by permission of the National Asthma and Respiratory Training Centre)

deconditioning of skeletal muscles and, in turn, increasing disability; COPD patients often report that the limiting factor to their exercise tolerance is tiredness in the legs rather than breathlessness. Avoiding exercise, as well as the fear that breathlessness invokes, leads to a general loss of confidence, sowing the seeds of social isolation and increasing dependence. Increasing inactivity and isolation further compound the problem and the patient is in a vicious circle that results in increasing dependence, disability and worsening quality of life (Figure 9.1.)

For many COPD patients the 'normal' irritations and stresses of everyday life are sufficient to induce breathlessness. The phenomenon of the 'emotional straitjacket' of advanced COPD is widely recognised.

- A passive dependent role may be adopted, in which the patient takes little part in family life.

- Patients feel they are a burden to their families.

- Frustration is often expressed as anger, usually directed at the family carer.

- Guilt at what is seen as a 'self-inflicted' disease is another common emotion.

- Resentment on the part of the carer at the restrictions this disease imposes on long-held plans for retirement may also be manifest.

- Self-destructive patterns of behaviour, such as a refusal to contemplate stopping smoking, are often seen.

- Self-esteem is frequently very low, and depression is common.

- Many patients refuse to exercise or will be restrained by an over-protective carer from exercising, even within their limited potential.

The aim of pulmonary rehabilitation is to break this vicious circle of increasing inactivity and breathlessness and to improve exercise capacity and functional ability.

The components of a hospital-based pulmonary rehabilitation programme

Pulmonary rehabilitation programmes usually consist of three main components:

- exercise training,
- education about the disease and its management,
- psychosocial support.

Exercise

Exercise (aerobic) training to recondition skeletal muscles and improve exercise endurance forms the cornerstone of most programmes. The amount of exercise prescribed is determined on an individual basis and is based either on a laboratory treadmill or cycle ergometer test or a field exercise test, such as the relatively simple shuttle walking test (see Chapter 5). The shuttle walking test is closely related to an individual's peak oxygen consumption (Vo_2 peak) and allows a reasonably accurate prescription of exercise. It has been suggested that, when there is no access to exercise-testing equipment, patients may be able to determine their own training regimen, based on their perception of breathlessness. A Borg scale (see Table 5.2) is often employed, and the patient is encouraged to exercise to between levels 3 and 5 (moderate to severe).

Most hospital-based programmes use cycling or walking for exercise endurance training. Generally, an attempt is made to prescribe a form of regular exercise that the patient will find easy to continue at home both during and after the rehabilitation programme. Walking and cycling are also activities that have some meaning for the patient in terms of their daily lives.

Exercises that train specific groups of muscles, such as the upper limb girdle muscles, are usually included in a training programme and are aimed at improving the patient's ability to perform particular tasks associated with daily living. In someone with COPD the accessory muscles of respiration may be used. Any activity that uses the same muscle groups, such as brushing the hair or carrying shopping, is likely to increase the breathlessness. Specific exercises for particular muscle groups may be of great benefit for patients with severe COPD, who may find aerobic exercise too demanding. The exercises are generally of the more gentle bend-and-stretch variety, but may still give good results in increasing functional ability.

The role of respiratory muscle training in pulmonary rehabilitation is debatable. Training the respiratory muscles for strength and endurance has been successful in healthy subjects and in patients with chronic airflow obstruction but evidence that such training produces clinically significant results is equivocal. Further research is awaited.

Hospital pulmonary rehabilitation programmes are generally multidisciplinary and do not consist of exercise training alone. The first hour of a session is usually devoted to an exercise routine and the second hour to educating the patient and family about the disease, its management and how to develop strategies to live with it (summarised in Table 9.1). Partners and carers are generally actively encouraged to attend. A carer's need for information and social support is often as great as, if not greater than, the patient's.

Table 9.1 Components of pulmonary rehabilitation

Exercise

Endurance (aerobic) training:
    Walking
    Cycling
Specific muscle groups (e.g. upper limb girdle)
?Respiratory muscle training (value debatable)

Education

The lungs in health and disease
Drug treatment
Self-management
Stopping smoking
Nutrition
Breathing control and sputum clearance
Relaxation techniques/coping strategies
Dealing with everyday activities
Financial support and benefits

Education and advice

People need basic information about the lungs in health and disease to help them understand the role of smoking in the development of COPD. Some centres exclude patients who continue to smoke but others will accept them and include smoking cessation in their education programme. There is certainly some logic to this approach. If smokers are excluded from rehabilitation, a low self-esteem – 'I'm not worth the trouble' – may well be reinforced. Joining a programme with other COPD sufferers who have successfully 'kicked the habit' may provide added incentive for an attempt to quit.

Advice is also given about the drug treatment of COPD and how to manage exacerbations effectively. Other professionals may be involved in giving additional education. For example:

■ Dieticians can provide valuable general advice on healthy eating; they are also available to provide specific advice to the overweight or underweight patient.

■ A physiotherapist can teach sputum clearance techniques and breathing control. Relaxation and coping skills are also valuable.

■ The occupational therapist can provide advice or equipment to help with activities of daily living.

■ The social worker may be able to give advice on benefits and financial matters.

Marital and sexual problems are common among these patients, so specialist help and advice may also be needed.

Psychosocial support

Many patients with advanced COPD are socially isolated. Pulmonary rehabilitation programmes can provide both patients and their partners/carers with valuable social contact. The support provided by group members can be enormous.

The setting of pulmonary rehabilitation and the personnel involved vary widely, depending very much on local circumstances. Some centres offer inpatient rehabilitation and in some areas home or primary-care-based programmes are available. Generally, a programme will consist of two or three sessions a week for six to eight weeks, combined with a programme of exercises the patient performs at home between sessions. The maintenance of improvement after a rehabilitation programme seems to be long-lasting but some sort of follow-up and after-care would probably be beneficial. Clearly, for this to be provided indefinitely in a hospital setting would be expensive and, it could be argued, might serve to undermine the philosophy of self-reliance that is engendered as part of the initial programme.

The provision of a 'training diary' or an occasional 'refresher' session is offered by some centres as a solution to the problem of continuing support. In others, patients 'graduate' from pulmonary rehabilitation to a patient support group. The British Lung Foundation's Breathe Easy groups provide an ideal forum for continuing social contact, support and encouragement. Some centres graduate less severely disabled patients to an 'exercise on prescription' group at local sports centres where they can still meet regularly, exercise and benefit from mutual support.

The role of the primary health care team

The provision of hospital-based rehabilitation programmes is far from uniform at present. The role of the primary health care team is:

- to select appropriate patients for referral where such schemes exist,

- to support and encourage patients undergoing rehabilitation, and

- to follow-up and provide continued encouragement for patients who have graduated from hospital programmes.

Before a referral for rehabilitation is considered, it should be ensured that the patient is on optimum therapy and that no further improvements with additional drug intervention can be achieved. It is also usual to refer patients in a period of clinical stability, although for those who have frequent exacerbations this may be difficult and referrals may be appropriate during a convalescent period. It is also important to consider whether the patient's disability is related solely to COPD or if there is a significant co-morbidity that will limit the effectiveness of rehabilitation. For example, a patient who has severe rheumatoid arthritis or ischaemic heart disease may be

Table 9.2 Patient selection

Motivated to improve

On optimal treatment and compliant with treatment

Increasing disability

Clinically stable

Able to exercise (caution with cardiac, orthopaedic or neurological problems)

unable to undertake the exercise component of the programme. However, some centres will accept such patients for the education component of the programme.

The selection of appropriate patients is crucial and is not based solely on clinical criteria (Table 9.2):

■ Current smokers might not be accepted, as discussed earlier. Some physicians consider that patients who are unable to stop smoking are unlikely to be able to make the lifestyle changes that are at the core of rehabilitation and are also unlikely to adhere to an exercise programme.

■ Difficulties with travel may mean that ambulance transport will have to be arranged.

■ If the patient is still working, there may be difficulties with attending all the sessions.

■ Perhaps the most important consideration of all is *the patient's motivation to improve.*

If your area includes people from ethnic minorities, there may be language and culture difficulties. However, it may be possible to gather a group of patients of the same ethnic origin and use an interpreter who can also advise on cultural aspects.

The fact that a patient is using oxygen is not generally a reason to exclude them from a rehabilitation programme, and neither is the severity of their condition. It could be argued that patients with severe disease stand to gain the most from rehabilitation.

Where there are no formal rehabilitation programmes, the primary health care team may need to be innovative and enlist whatever services are available locally. A community physiotherapist, particularly if they have a respiratory interest, may be a useful resource. Leaflets containing information about suitable gentle exercises and breathing control are available from the British Lung Foundation (see 'Useful address' at the end of this chapter). Patients need to be reassured that getting breathless when exercising will not cause any further damage to their lungs, and they should all be encouraged to keep active and take some form of regular exercise. A daily walk or regular stair climbing fit well with everyday life and may be more likely to be adhered to on a regular basis than a series of exercises that the patient sees as bearing little relation to their normal activities.

Rehabilitation may be unfamiliar territory for the primary care team. When advising about exercise there can be understandable concerns if the patient also suffers from ischaemic heart disease. It may be better, therefore, to start with an 'uncomplicated' patient and to keep advice simple and practical. The family focus of primary care and its ability to provide long-term follow-up and care make it an ideal setting for the education, follow-up and encouragement of COPD patients and their families.

Finally, when you are encouraging someone to exercise, the type is perhaps less important than its regularity. It is important not to deter patients with too rigid or complicated an exercise regimen. The essence is to encourage, to reassure that they will do themselves no harm and, perhaps most important of all, to persuade them that they are worth the effort.

Further reading

GOLDSTEIN RS, GORT EH, STUBBING D, AVENDANO MA, GUYATT GH (1994) Randomised controlled trial of respiratory rehabilitation. *Lancet* **344**: 1394–7

HODGKIN JE (1990) Pulmonary rehabilitation. *Clinics in Chest Medicine* **11**: 447–60

LACASSE Y, WONG E, GUYATT GH et al. (1996) Meta-analysis of respiratory rehabilitation in chronic obstructive pulmonary disease. *Lancet* **348**: 1115–89

MORGAN M, SINGH S (1997) *Practical Pulmonary Rehabilitation.* Chapman and Hall Medical, London.

NIEDERMAN MS, CLEMENTE PH, FEIN AM et al. (1991) Benefits of a multidisciplinary pulmonary rehabilitation program. Improvements are independent of lung function. *Chest* **99**: 798–804

Reiss AL, Kaplan RM, Limberg TM, Prewitt LM (1995) Effects of pulmonary rehabilitation on physiologic and psychosocial outcomes in patients with chronic obstructive pulmonary disease. *Annals of Internal Medicine* **122**: 823–32

Singh SJ, Morgan MDL, Hardman AE et al. (1994) Comparison of oxygen uptake during a conventional treadmill test and the shuttle walking test in chronic airflow limitation. *European Respiratory Journal* **7**: 2016–20

Toshima MT, Kaplan RM, Reiss AL (1990) Experimental evaluation of rehabilitation in chronic obstructive pulmonary disease: short-term effects on exercise endurance and health status. *Health Psychology* **93**: 237–52

Wijkstra PJ, Ten Vergert EM, Van Altena R et al. (1990) Long term benefits of rehabilitation at home on quality of life and exercise tolerance in patients with chronic obstructive pulmonary disease. *Thorax* **50**: 824–8

Useful address

Breathe Easy
British Lung Foundation
78 Hatton Garden
London EC1N 8LD
Tel: 020 7831 5831

10 | Other forms of therapy

Main points

Oxygen

1 Long-term oxygen therapy (LTOT) improves breathlessness and survival in severe COPD.

2 To be effective, LTOT must be administered for at least 15 hours per day.

3 The most cost-effective way of administering oxygen over long periods is by oxygen concentrator. This also allows the patient much greater mobility around the home while still receiving oxygen.

4 Ambulatory oxygen is available from small cylinders but these last only two hours and are not very practical.

5 Patients with severe COPD need specialist advice before flying or travelling to high altitude.

Surgery

1 The surgical removal of large bullae may significantly improve lung function and symptoms.

2 Surgery to reduce lung volume is gaining in popularity but should be performed only in specialist centres and with careful patient selection. It has an operative mortality of 1–3% but can produce good clinical improvements.

3 Lung transplants are usually performed on younger patients (below 50 years) with alpha-1 antitrypsin deficiency emphysema.

Vaccination

1 Vaccination annually against influenza is recommended.

2 The Department of Health recommends pneumococcal vaccination for patients with COPD.

Nutrition

1 Diets rich in antioxidants (e.g. fresh fruit and vegetables) may help to slow the progress of COPD.

2 Obese patients should be vigorously encouraged to lose weight, which will reduce breathlessness and improve mobility.

3 Many patients with advanced emphysema are underweight and have extensive muscle wasting. The mechanism is not certain but inflammatory cytokines may have a role.

4 Patients with muscle wasting need advice on an appropriate diet.

5 The life expectancy is worse for COPD patients who are underweight and have muscle wasting.

Oxygen therapy

Patients with severe COPD who are in chronic respiratory failure benefit from oxygen, but it has to be given over long periods every day. The aims of long-term oxygen therapy (LTOT) are thus quite different from the short-term use of oxygen in hospital for patients with acute exacerbations.

At sea level the atmosphere contains around 21% oxygen. LTOT aims to increase the concentration of oxygen in inhaled air to around 30%. This level generally provides the best tissue oxygenation without increasing the arterial carbon dioxide and worsening the respiratory failure. The results of two placebo-controlled trials of LTOT revealed:

- improved survival,

- reduced polycythaemia,

- no progression of pulmonary hypertension,

- slightly improved health status.

The first of these trials, conducted by the Medical Research Council (MRC), showed that 15 hours of oxygen per day increased five-year survival from 25% to 41%. The second trial – the Nocturnal Oxygen Therapy Trial (NOTT) – demonstrated that continuous oxygen (mean use of 17.7 hours per day) was beneficial, but that use for only 12 hours per day conferred no benefit.

A further study of patients using 15 hours of oxygen per day showed that, although five-year survival was 62%, this had dropped to only 26% at ten years. Why some patients do better than others is incompletely understood. Generally, the patients who obtained most benefit from LTOT had:

- a higher $Paco_2$,

- a higher packed cell volume (haematocrit),

- a higher pulmonary pressure,

- a lower FVC.

A good prognostic indicator was a fall in pulmonary artery pressure of more than 5mmHg over 24 hours when oxygen was given.

The clinical benefits of LTOT, apart from increased life expectancy, are an increase in exercise tolerance and reduced breathlessness. Whether LTOT improves health status is debatable. A striking finding in patients being considered for LTOT is the very high level of emotional and mood disturbance. These patients have severe disease: depression is thus very common and low self-esteem almost universal. Whilst the NOTT study did not show any change in health status on oxygen, the results from other studies have indicated improvement in mood and depression indices, well-being and breathlessness scores, exercise tolerance and sleep patterns. Generally, physicians with extensive experience of LTOT are favourably impressed with the improvements in quality of life that these patients can achieve.

Who should receive LTOT?

In general, patients considered for LTOT:

- have severe COPD,

- are hypoxic,

- have evidence of right ventricular strain and peripheral oedema.

It is important that patients are assessed by a respiratory physician. Measurements of lung function and arterial blood gases are needed. If the criteria outlined below are met, the patient needs a trial of oxygen in hospital with further measurement of blood gases to determine what concentration of oxygen is required to correct the hypoxia without causing an undue increase in the level of carbon dioxide. It is essential that arterial blood gases for assessment for LTOT are taken when the patient has been clinically stable for at least a month. Drug therapy should be optimised; steroid trials should have been performed and the possibility of further benefit from increased bronchodilator doses or improved delivery systems investigated. Patients *must* have stopped smoking: smoking in the presence of oxygen constitutes an explosive hazard, and there is evidence that LTOT has no benefit for patients who continue to smoke.

Although the decision to refer a patient for oxygen therapy is best made on clinical grounds together with the spirometry, pulse oximetry may be a useful screening tool in general practice. If the oxygen saturation is less than 92% when the patient is stable, referral for blood gases and further investigation is likely to be needed.

Clinical criteria for LTOT

- FEV_1 less than 1.5 litres,

- arterial hypoxia (Pao_2 less than7.3kPa), with or without hypercapnia,

- evidence of peripheral oedema and pulmonary hypertension, or nocturnal hypoxia,

- non-smoker.

Oxygen should correct the blood gases to an arterial oxygen tension

(Pao_2) greater than 8kPa, without causing a rise in arterial carbon dioxide ($Paco_2$) that significantly increases the level of respiratory failure.

Oxygen concentrators?

In England, Wales and Northern Ireland the patient's GP will be asked to prescribe an oxygen concentrator. In Scotland, concentrators are prescribed by the respiratory physician.

To confer any benefit, LTOT must be used for at least 15 hours per day. This is best achieved using an oxygen concentrator with nasal prongs, at a flow rate of either 2 or 4 litres per minute. The flow rate is determined during the hospital trial and must be stipulated on the prescription for the concentrator. The concentrator is prescribed on a standard FP10 form, which is given to the patient. It should contain the following information.

- oxygen concentrator,

- flow rate in litres per minute,

- number of hours per day it should be used,

- back-up oxygen cylinder (if required).

Information on the regional suppliers of concentrators in the UK can be found in the *British National Formulary* (*BNF*). The regional supplier will deliver and install the concentrator and maintain it regularly. The patient is regularly supplied with replacement nasal prongs and tubing. The concentrator contains a meter for recording the number of hours it has been used. This allows the electricity costs to be reimbursed direct to the patient and compliance to be assessed. All regional oxygen supply companies have a 24-hour call-out service in case the concentrator breaks down.

Follow-up blood gas measurement should be performed after six months of treatment. Increasingly, the specialist respiratory nurse at the local chest unit provides regular follow-up and gives the patient and their carers valuable psychological and social support.

Patients using concentrators occasionally have problems with drying of the nasal mucosa and soreness from the nasal prongs. A humidifier can be added into the system but great care is needed with its maintenance to prevent infection. Water-based creams such as E45 around the nostrils may reduce soreness. Using nasal prongs can also cause soreness around the ears and across the cheeks, so the oxygen tubing may need to be padded.

Cost/benefit

The use of domestic size oxygen cylinders (size F) for 15 hours per day costs around £6,500 per year. The cost of a concentrator is considerably less at £1,500, plus about £80 per month for maintenance and £20 per month for electricity, the cost of which is refunded to the patient. The major expense of the concentrator is the installation. Concentrators are very much more convenient for the patient to use and enable greater mobility around the home. A size F cylinder needs to be changed every 11 hours or so, so spare cylinders must be ordered, delivered and stored. It is not possible to fit long lengths of tubing to a cylinder and the patient is effectively 'chained' to the oxygen source. Any benefits in improved exercise tolerance are therefore likely to be undermined. In contrast, up to 50 metres of tubing can be attached to a concentrator, allowing the patient a considerable degree of mobility around the home.

LTOT prolongs life and has some benefits in health status. A French survey of 13,500 patients using LTOT found that 55% of them were able to wash unaided. However, 25% never left their homes and 25% never went on holiday. It is possible that portable oxygen systems might improve this situation.

Ambulatory oxygen therapy

This form of therapy can improve exercise tolerance and lessen breathlessness, encouraging patients to leave their homes and lead a fuller life. It can be combined with LTOT. However, the only currently available form of ambulatory oxygen that can be prescribed is the small, portable PD cylinder, which provides only 2 hours of oxygen at 2 litres per minute. Oxygen conservation devices, such as the Oxylite, can double the life of a PD cylinder, but none of these devices is currently available on prescription. These limitations severely restrict the potential use of ambulatory oxygen in the UK.

Occasional oxygen use by cylinder

Many patients are prescribed oxygen to be used as required when breathless, or to enable them to perform activities around the house more easily. There have been no clinical studies of this role of oxygen but, anecdotally, patients often find it beneficial. There are no recommendations for such prescribing in the BTS Guidelines. Patients prescribed oxygen for use in this way might also fit the criteria for LTOT, and consideration should be given for specialist assessment.

Travel and flying

Patients with severe COPD will often require advice about travel, particularly if flying is involved. Aircraft cabin pressures are equivalent to 5,000–8,000 feet above sea level, which reduces the ambient oxygen pressure to 15–18kPa. In a healthy individual this will reduce mean arterial oxygen from 12kPa to 8.7kPa, with a relatively insignificant drop in oxygen saturation from 96% to 90%. In patients with severe lung disease and hypoxia this reduction in ambient oxygen pressure is likely to cause a potentially hazardous drop in arterial oxygen levels unless they are given supplemental oxygen during the flight.

It has been suggested that for a patient to be safe to fly:

■ the FEV_1 should be in excess of 25% of the predicted value,

■ the Pao_2 should be greater than 6.7kPa,

■ there should be no hypercapnia.

Oxygen can be arranged on most scheduled flights by prior arrangement, but the cost can vary from nothing at all to £100 per flight, depending on the airline.

Patients with recent pneumothorax or emphysematous bullae may also be at increased risk of spontaneous pneumothorax while flying. Travel by land or sea is usually less of a problem.

If there is any doubt about the advisability of air travel, patients should be referred for assessment by a respiratory physician. Some centres can perform a hypoxic challenge by giving patients air with reduced oxygen levels by cylinder in order to assess their response to the reduced oxygen levels they are likely to experience during a flight.

Surgery

Treatment of emphysematous bullae

A small proportion of COPD patients may develop large cyst-like spaces – bullae – in the lung. These tend to compress the more normal areas of lung, thus reducing their ability to function efficiently. Large bullae can form in relatively normal lung or with any degree of emphysema. It is not clear how bullae originate but it is most likely that an area of local lung degeneration acts as the focus for an enlarging space. Surgery in such cases can significantly improve symptoms and function.

The symptoms produced by bullae are similar to those from the associated underlying emphysema. They can, however, usually be readily detected on a routine chest x-ray. Rarely, they can present as a pneumothorax. Before surgery is considered, there must be careful specialist physiological assessment and anatomical imaging of the bullae and surrounding lung with CT scanning. The best results are usually obtained in younger patients with large bullae and lesser degrees of airflow obstruction. The degree of emphysema in the surrounding lung is an important determinant of the success of this procedure.

There are a number of surgical approaches, ranging from thoracotomy to a laser technique via a thoracoscope. The aim is to obliterate the abnormal space and restore the elastic integrity of the lung, allowing the compressed areas of the lung to re-expand. Benefits from the surgery are usually felt almost immediately, and the improvement in lung function and symptoms seems to be maintained. Deterioration after the surgery seems to follow the standard course for a patient with emphysema. Operative mortality is low and should decrease further as the preoperative assessment procedures to screen out unsuitable patients improve.

Surgery to reduce lung volume

Lung volume reduction surgery is a relatively new technique. It was developed in the USA but is gaining in popularity in the UK. The operation is performed through a sternal split and involves one or both lungs. The aim is to remove 20–30% of the most distended emphysematous parts of the lungs. The lungs are then stapled and sutured to prevent air leaks. Complications are not uncommon, particularly relating to air leaks. Operative mortality is, at present, 1–3% depending on the centre. Careful preoperative assessment seems to be the key to success.

Lung volume reduction particularly reduces residual volume, improving vital capacity by 20–40%. FEV_1 can increase by between 20% and 80%, and the six-minute walking distance may improve by 30%. Longer term follow-up shows that the peak effect seems to occur at six to eight months following surgery, after which there is a slow decline. However, after two years most patients will still have better lung function than they had before the surgery.

This surgical technique is still in its infancy and many more carefully controlled studies are needed to fully evaluate its usefulness.

Lung transplant

Single lung transplant is the favoured option for emphysema, although double lung transplant procedures can be performed. The operation is generally straightforward and the results are deemed to be excellent. FEV_1 is usually restored to 50% of the predicted value. Lung transplantation is usually offered only to patients under 50 years of age, so the procedure is a likely option for alpha-1 anti-trypsin deficiency emphysema, which presents in this young age group. Generally it is considered only for patients with a life expectancy of less than 18 months. UK survival figures are 60% at three years.

The main drawbacks are related to tissue rejection and immuno-suppressant therapy. A late and serious complication is the development of obliterative bronchiolitis, which occurs in 30% of patients surviving five years. Unfortunately, this widespread inflammatory fibrotic condition of the small airways is frequently fatal at between six and twelve months.

Vaccinations

Influenza

Vaccination against influenza is recommended for all elderly patients, and has reduced mortality by 70% in this group. It is also indicated for people with a range of chronic diseases, including COPD, and for anyone with decreased immunity. There have been no trials of its efficacy specifically in COPD but, by inference from the data relating to elderly people, there ought to be benefits from regular annual vaccination.

Pneumococcus

Streptococcus pneumoniae is the commonest cause of community-acquired pneumonia. Pneumococcal infection is more common in adults over 50 years; in people over 65 years the risk of infection increases by two- to fivefold. The Department of Health includes COPD patients in its at-risk groups for pneumococcal vaccination. Immunisation should be with the polyvalent vaccine, which is a single injection. Immunocompromised or splenectomised patients should be given booster injections every five years.

There are no controlled studies of the effectiveness of this vaccine in COPD, although an evaluation from the USA concluded that the vaccination of people over 65 years is cost saving.

Nutrition

There is some epidemiological evidence suggesting that diets rich in fresh fruit and vegetables are beneficial in slowing the progression of COPD. Such diets are also, of course, valuable in reducing the risk of coronary artery disease and some cancers. It is thought that the high levels of antioxidants in vitamins C and E have a protective effect on lung tissue. However, a study with vitamin E supplements failed to find any significant benefit compared with a placebo. It is also thought that some natural fish oils may protect the lungs through antioxidant enhancement, but scientific evidence for this is lacking.

Obesity

COPD patients who are overweight are likely to have greater impairment of activity and will experience a greater degree of breathlessness than patients of a normal weight. This in turn causes them to lead a more sedentary existence and have a worsened quality of life. You should encourage overweight patients to lose weight as well as to get regular exercise. (See also Chapter 9.)

Malnutrition and muscle wasting

A low body mass index (BMI) and loss of lean muscle mass are common in COPD, especially when emphysema is the predominant pathological problem. Weight loss is a poor prognostic sign and a low BMI increases the risk of death from COPD.

The cause of weight loss in emphysema is complex and poorly understood. It used to be thought that the chronically increased work of breathing, coupled with difficulties in shopping, preparing food and eating when constantly breathless, caused a negative energy balance and, thus, weight loss. This is now thought not to be the sole cause as, in addition to weight loss, most people with COPD have peripheral muscle weakness linked to loss of muscle mass. It has been discovered that there are systemic inflammatory processes and changes in muscle metabolism in these patients.

Raised levels of certain cytokines, including interleukin 8 (IL-8) and tumour necrosis factor alpha (TNF-α), have been found, and these seem likely to have an important role in causing loss of muscle mass. Increased levels of cytokines may be a response to low levels of oxygen in the tissues (tissue hypoxia), resulting from the destruction of alveoli. This might help to explain why weight loss occurs in some patients with comparatively minor FEV_1 impairment and why patients with chronic bronchitis do not seem to have comparable tissue hypoxia and weight loss.

It should be remembered that loss of muscle mass is also a consequence of the muscle deconditioning that occurs from lack of activity.

It is possible – though difficult – to treat and partially reverse this weight loss. Increased exercise, particularly through a programme of pulmonary rehabilitation, coupled with nutritional supplements and, rarely, anabolic steroids have increased both weight and muscle mass. This may result in a small increase in survival rate for patients who gain weight. Non-steroidal anti-inflammatory drugs (NSAIDs) have been used to block the action of the cytokines that may be involved in causing weight loss in patients with terminal cancer, but this does not seem to have been tried in COPD.

Breathlessness can make the very act of eating tiring. Eating can also induce greater breathlessness. Practical advice to patients includes eating small but frequent high-calorie meals. Fish is more digestible than meat and requires less effort to chew. Pureed vegetables and soups also require less effort to consume. Referral to a dietician may be helpful for some patients.

Exercise

Exercise is an important part of the management of COPD, and is discussed in detail in Chapter 9. Regular exercise is helpful both physically and psychologically, and encourages patients to lead a more normal social life. Encourage patients to regularly walk to the point of breathlessness. Explain that regular walking, pushing themselves a little further each day, will help improve physical fitness. They need reassurance that breathlessness in these circumstances will do no harm to their heart or lungs and is, in fact, positively beneficial. Repeating these positive messages at follow-up visits is helpful.

Social and psychological issues

Many patients with more severe COPD are clinically anxious or depressed. They may feel embarrassed by their breathlessness or inability to exercise, and therefore may tend not to go out and socialise. They may feel guilty about their inability to perform jobs around the house and garden. Impaired activity levels affect both the patient and their partner, family and carers, and can reduce their ability to socialise, take holidays and enjoy a normal life.

Counselling and encouragement to obtain benefits may help to improve health status. The local Citizens Advice Bureau and the Benefits Agency may be able to help with information about entitlement to state benefits and how to apply for them. Obtaining an Orange Badge (becoming a Blue Badge in 2000) – which permits car parking in many restricted areas – may help with mobility and enable patients to get out more. Local voluntary organisations may also be able to help both patients and carers in a wide range of activities, including respite care.

Depression should be treated with standard forms of therapy where indicated. Care should be taken, however, not to prescribe medication that might depress the respiratory drive. Small amounts of alcohol are acceptable and, for people with severe COPD who have difficulty sleeping, may be preferable to sleeping pills.

Severe breathlessness and terminal disease

In end-stage COPD, breathlessness may be so severe that eating and talking become difficult and life is distressing for both patient and carer. Bronchodilators in high doses are the first line of therapy, either by large volume spacer or by nebuliser. Oral prednisolone in doses up to 40mg per day may produce initial improvement, but the benefit is usually small. Oxygen in short bursts from a cylinder is often prescribed.

Other drugs that reduce anxiety or induce a sense of well-being, such as diazepam, morphine or dihydrocodeine, have been used in the terminal stages but with little reported benefit. Because they all have depressant effects on the respiratory drive, they must be used with great caution. Advice should be sought from a specialist in terminal and palliative care.

Further reading

Oxygen therapy

Cooper CB, Waterhouse J, Howard P (1987) Twelve year clinical study of patients with chronic hypoxic cor pulmonale given long-term oxygen therapy. *Thorax* **42**: 105–10

Cooper CB (1995) Domiciliary oxygen therapy. In: Calverley PMA, Pride NB (eds) *Chronic Obstructive Lung Disease*. Chapman and Hall, London; 495–526

Dilworth JP, Higgs CMB, Jones PA et al. (1990) Acceptability of oxygen concentrators; the patients' view. *British Journal of General Practice* **40**: 415–17

Lahdensuo A, Ojanen M, Ahonen A et al. (1989) Psychological effects of continuous oxygen therapy in hypoxic chronic obstructive pulmonary disease patients. *European Respiratory Journal* **2**: 977–80

Nocturnal Oxygen Therapy Trial Group (1980) Continuous or nocturnal oxygen therapy in hypoxic chronic obstructive lung disease. *Annals of Internal Medicine* **93**: 391–8

Medical Research Council Oxygen Working Party (1981) Report. Long-term domiciliary oxygen therapy in chronic hypoxic cor pulmonale complicating chronic bronchitis and emphysema. *Lancet* **1**: 681–6

ROBERTS CM, FRANKLIN J, O'NEILL R et al. (1998) Screening patients in general practice with COPD for long term domiciliary oxygen requirement using pulse oximetry. *Respiratory Medicine* **92**: 1265–8

WALTERS MI, EDWARDS PR, WATERHOUSE JC, HOWARD P (1993) Long term domiciliary oxygen therapy in chronic obstructive pulmonary disease. *Thorax* **48**: 1170–7

Surgery

BRENNER M, MCKENNA RJ, GELB AF et al. (1998) Rate of FEV₁ change following lung reduction surgery. *Chest* **113**: 652–9

McGRAW L (1997) Lung volume reduction surgery: an overview. *Heart and Lung* **26**: 131–7

O'BRIEN GM, CRINER GJ (1998) Surgery for severe COPD. Lung volume reduction and lung transplantation. *Postgraduate Medical Journal* **103**: 179–94

Nutrition

SCHOLS AMWJ, SLANGEN J, VOLOVICS L et al. (1998) Weight loss is a reversible factor in the prognosis of chronic obstructive pulmonary disease. *American Journal of Respiratory and Critical Care Medicine* **157**: 1791–7

SRIDHAR MK (1995) Why do patients with emphysema lose weight? *Lancet* **345**: 1190–1

Depression and psychosocial issues

DUDLEY DL, GLASER EM, JORGENSON BN et al. (1980) Psychosocial concomitants to rehabilitation in obstructive pulmonary disease. *Chest* **77**: 41

Acute exacerbations and referral to hospital

Main points

1 Exacerbations of symptoms are common, the frequency increasing with more severe levels of COPD. They tend to occur more often in winter.

2 Exacerbations may be infective, characterised by increasing sputum volume, sputum purulence and breathlessness; or they may be related to changes in airflow obstruction, with increased breathlessness, wheeze and cough.

3 Treatment may include:
   – increased bronchodilators,
   – antibiotics,
   – a course of oral corticosteroids for one to two weeks.

4 The decision to manage the exacerbation at home or admit the patient to hospital is based on a list of clinical and social factors summarised in Table 11.1.

5 A prolonged worsening of symptoms should raise the suspicion of other diagnoses (e.g. lung cancer) and lead to further investigation such as chest x-ray and possible referral to hospital.

6 There may be other causes of persistent cough, such as chronic nasal catarrh and postnasal drip. These should be investigated and treated accordingly.

7 Plans for COPD patient self-management have not yet been developed. Advice on the use of antibiotics and oral steroids may help with earlier treatment of exacerbations.

8 The suspicion of respiratory failure in exacerbations should lead to hospital admission and measurement of arterial blood gases.

9 Criteria for referral to a specialist are listed in Table 11.2.

Many patients with moderate or severe levels of COPD experience regular exacerbations of their symptoms, particularly during the winter. Most exacerbations can be managed in the community but more symptomatic patients, or those whose social circumstances are poor, are likely to need admission to hospital.

Common symptoms of exacerbations are:

- increases in sputum purulence (white sputum becoming yellow or green),

- increases in sputum volume,

- increased breathlessness, wheeze and chest tightness,

- sometimes, fluid retention with ankle swelling.

Exacerbations are broadly of two kinds:

- an infection with change in sputum colour and possibly fever,

- changes in lung mechanics and airflow obstruction where patients experience greater breathlessness, wheeze and chest tightness but without evidence of infection.

Both sets of symptoms may occur together. The cause of worsening lung function is frequently not clear. COPD patients often report brief worsening of symptoms on days that are cold, damp or windy but measured lung function on such occasions usually remains unchanged.

Increasing or worsening symptoms may also be caused by other disease processes, and the following should be considered from the history and examination:

- pneumonia,

- pneumothorax,

- pulmonary oedema,

- pulmonary embolism,

- lung cancer,

- upper airway obstruction or foreign body.

Management of the acute exacerbation

Clinical examination during an acute exacerbation is likely to reveal a patient who is breathless, wheezy and coughing, and whose PEF is lower than usual. They may also be cyanosed and have peripheral oedema. A patient who is drowsy, dehydrated or confused is usually in significant respiratory failure and will need urgent admission to hospital. It is helpful to know the patient's usual clinical state so that comparisons can be made. An assessment of the social circumstances and the patient's ability to cope at home are as important as the clinical assessment when making the important decision about whether to manage them at home or to admit them to hospital. The BTS *COPD Guidelines* outlined in Table 11.1 give some pointers.

Treatment in the community

Antibiotics

If the symptoms are suggestive of an infection, it is common practice for antibiotics to be prescribed. Criteria for using antibiotics should include two or more of the following:

- purulent sputum,
- increased sputum volume,
- increased breathlessness.

The most common pathogens are *Haemophilus influenzae, Streptococcus pneumoniae* and *Moraxella catarrhalis*. Occasionally, *Chlamydia pneumoniae* is found. The most appropriate antibiotic should follow local microbiology guidelines but standard antibiotics such as amoxycillin, erythromycin and tetracycline, all for seven days, are normally satisfactory. Sputum culture is not usually indicated.

Bronchodilators

For both infective and non-infective exacerbations, the dose of beta-agonist and/or anticholinergic inhaled bronchodilators should be

Table 11.1 Deciding whether to treat an acute exacerbation at home or in hospital

	Treat at home	Treat in hospital
Able to cope at home	Yes	No
Breathlessness	Mild	Severe
General condition	Good	Poor, deteriorating
Level of activity	Good	Poor, confined to bed
Cyanosis	No	Yes
Worsening peripheral oedema	No	Yes
Level of consciousness	Normal	Impaired
Already receiving LTOT	No	Yes
Social circumstances	Good	Living alone/not coping
Acute confusion	No	Yes
Rapid rate of onset	No	Yes
Also available at hospital		
Changes on the chest x-ray	No	Present
Arterial pH level	> 7.35	< 7.35
Arterial Pao$_2$	> 7kPa	< 7kPa

The more referral indicators that are present, the more likely the need for admission to hospital.

increased, or started four-hourly if the patient is not already taking a bronchodilator. A short course of oral beta-agonist may be helpful in patients who have difficulty using inhaled medication, but care should be taken if there are coexisting diseases such as angina, particularly in elderly people. Multiple doses of inhaled broncho-dilators are safe and can be administered to very breathless patients via a large volume spacer. It is rare that a nebuliser is needed for acute attacks.

Oral corticosteroids

Steroids may be helpful in exacerbations not caused by infection, where lung function has deteriorated significantly. They may also be added to antibiotics for an infection accompanied by marked wheeze and breathlessness. A course of prednisolone 30mg per day is given for seven days and is usually then discontinued unless the patient has failed to recover fully.

Patients already on long-term oral steroids should have the dose increased to 30–40mg per day; on recovery the dose should be reduced over several weeks back to the previous baseline level. Patients usually respond well to corticosteroids in exacerbations related to increased airflow obstruction but there are very few published clinical studies to support this (see also Chapter 8).

Follow-up

Exacerbations treated in the community normally respond well to the therapy outlined above. Patients who fail to respond need further examination and review. An important differential diagnosis to exclude in a patient who is slow in responding is lung cancer. If this is suspected, a chest x-ray should be performed and consideration given to referral to a respiratory specialist.

Follow-up is a good opportunity to assess the patient's clinical state, treatment and social circumstances and also to reiterate messages about smoking, weight loss and exercise.

Recurrent exacerbations

Someone with severe COPD may have many exacerbations in a year. The presence of persistent purulent sputum, perhaps with inspiratory coarse crackles – particularly at the lung bases – may suggest a diagnosis of bronchiectasis. Alternatively, and fairly rarely, patients may have an immune deficiency syndrome or abnormality of cilial function (immotile cilia syndrome).

Persistent nasal catarrh and postnasal drip can cause a productive cough. Treating the nose with decongestants and/or a course of betamethasone and neomycin nose drops, given with the correct technique, may clear the nose and reduce the cough.

Self-management

There are not yet any specific self-management schemes for COPD like those for asthma. For patients who have regular infective exacerbations it is sensible to provide emergency standby supplies of an appropriate antibiotic, which they can take immediately if their sputum increases in volume and becomes purulent.

Similarly, if patients have previously benefited from courses of oral prednisolone, it is reasonable to provide them with an emergency supply to take if there is a marked worsening of breathlessness and wheeze over a 24-hour period. Such patients might monitor their PEF at home but there is no hard evidence to indicate the value of this.

Respiratory failure

Respiratory failure is a clinical state characterised by severe hypoxia (Pao_2 less than 7.3kPa), with or without accompanying hypercapnia. The diagnosis is made by measurement of arterial blood gases.

Respiratory failure may accompany exacerbations of COPD. Clinical suspicion of hypoxia includes cyanosis and breathlessness. A raised level of arterial carbon dioxide causes symptoms of central nervous system depression with drowsiness, coma, confusion and mood change. There may also be symptoms of tremor and flap of the hands, muscle jerks and convulsions. The vasodilator effect of raised carbon dioxide results in a bounding pulse, flushed skin and headache, sometimes related to papilloedema. Such patients will always need urgent admission to hospital.

Great care must be taken with oxygen therapy on the way to hospital. Inspired oxygen of 28% via Venturi mask or 2 litres per minute via nasal cannula is the maximum that is safe in an ambulance or at home. Higher levels of inspired oxygen can remove hypoxic respiratory drive and lead to respiratory arrest.

Treatment of associated conditions

Patients with severe COPD frequently develop pulmonary hypertension and cor pulmonale, usually presenting as peripheral oedema. The addition of diuretics and possibly an ACE inhibitor is indicated in patients with:

- peripheral oedema,
- a raised jugular venous pressure, and
- gallop heart rhythm.

There is no effective therapy for pulmonary hypertension alone but patients with cor pulmonale and right heart failure may benefit from long-term oxygen therapy (LTOT).

Consideration of specialist referral

The indications for specialist referral include:

- to make a diagnosis,
- to perform spirometry:
- to exclude other possible diagnoses such as lung cancer,
- to assess for oxygen therapy or long-term nebuliser treatment,
- to offer special advice to younger patients with alpha-1 antitrypsin deficiency.

The indications for specialist referral as set out in the BTS Guidelines are listed in Table 11.2

Table 11.2 Indications for specialist referral

Reason	Purpose
Therapeutic advice	
Suspected severe COPD	Confirm diagnosis and optimise therapy
Onset of cor pulmonale	Confirm diagnosis and optimise therapy
Assessment for oxygen therapy	Optimise therapy and measure blood gases
Assessment for nebuliser therapy	Exclude inappropriate prescriptions
Assessment for oral corticosteroids	Justify need for long-term treatment or to supervise withdrawal
Bullous lung disease	Identify candidates for surgery
A rapid decline in FEV_1	Encourage early intervention
Diagnostic advice	
Aged under 40 years or a family history of alpha-1 antitrypsin deficiency	Identify alpha-1 antitrypsin deficiency; consider therapy and screen family
Uncertain diagnosis	Make a diagnosis
Symptoms disproportionate to lung function deficit	Look for other explanations
Frequent infections	Exclude bronchiectasis

12 | Drug therapy of the future

Main points

1 Much research is in progress, looking for new treatments for COPD. The most promising therapies are focused on ways to prevent or block inflammatory changes, mediators and proteolytic enzymes.

2 An antidepressant drug, bupropion, that will help people to stop smoking should be available soon.

3 A promising new long-acting anticholinergic inhaled bronchodilator, tiotropium, will be available in the next few years.

4 Antioxidant therapy, either naturally with fruit and vegetables or with specific agents, may help slow the rate of progression of COPD.

One of the problems with writing books is that they are often out of date by the time they are published. This chapter is therefore confined to:

- therapy that is likely to appear in the next few years and be relevant and available to primary care,

- active research that is taking place along potentially beneficial lines.

Stopping smoking

Only 20–30% of patients are able to quit smoking (see Chapter 6). So far, nicotine replacement therapy has been the most effective way of enhancing the quit rate but some patients remain addicted to the nicotine product and there may be a risk of cardiovascular side-effects. An antidepressant tablet, bupropion (Zyban), with noradrenergic activity in the brain, has been shown to increase smoking cessation rates markedly. The drug is licensed in the USA and may appear soon in the UK.

Anticholinergic bronchodilators

The most promising new agent is an inhaled anticholinergic drug called tiotropium. It bonds well to the muscarinic, parasympathetic receptors in the lungs and remains attached to them for long periods, which results in long-term bronchodilation. The reports of studies with COPD patients indicate that its duration of action is over 24 hours, suggesting the feasibility of once-daily dosage. Tiotropium is likely to be available by 2001.

Anti-inflammatory therapies

Increasingly, the design of new drugs is geared towards the pathological changes that are observed in disease processes. Inflammatory changes are found in the airways of people with chronic bronchitis and, to some extent, the terminal airways of patients with emphysema. There are increases in the number of inflammatory cells, such as neutrophils, T-lymphocytes and alveolar macrophages.

Corticosteroids have only a modest effect, and over 80% of patients with COPD have no significant response to a formal oral steroid challenge test. Therefore other means of blocking the inflammatory process are being explored.

Leukotriene antagonists have been launched recently and have had a beneficial role in asthma. There have, as yet, been no trials of these agents in COPD but it is unlikely that the currently available drugs that block the leukotriene receptors will have a major role. However, leukotriene LTB4 is a potent stimulator of neutrophils, and its levels are increased in the sputum of COPD patients. Trials are currently in progress with selective LTB4 inhibitors, which may be useful in reducing sputum production and cough in COPD.

Another avenue of research is the development of agents that block some of the important family of enzymes called phosphodiesterases (PDEs). Theophyllines are thought to act in this way. Phosphodiesterases break down cyclic adenosine monophosphate (cyclic AMP), which has a crucial role in bronchodilation and in reducing many parts of the inflammatory cascade, especially relating to neutrophils. By blocking this enzyme, more cyclic AMP is available to promote beneficial actions in the airways. Clinical trials of the bronchodilator and anti-inflammatory effects of PDE4 inhibitors in COPD have just begun.

Antiproteases

There is evidence to suggest that one of the major factors in the development of lung damage and emphysema in COPD is over-activity of proteolytic enzymes released from neutrophils and macrophages. The enhanced cellular breakdown may be related to more enzyme release or decreased protective mechanisms, as in alpha-1 antitrypsin deficiency. Neutrophil elastase inhibitors have been developed but are awaiting clinical trials.

Alpha-1 antitrypsin

The genetically inherited homozygous deficiency of the antiprotease protein alpha-1 antitrypsin leads to the development of emphysema in the third decade of life. Various clinical trials have attempted to replace alpha-1 antitrypsin but the results have generally been disappointing. Alpha-1 antitrypsin can be extracted from plasma but the cost is high. A trial in the USA using weekly intravenous alpha-1 antitrypsin failed to halt the decline in lung function. A nebulised formulation – also very expensive – has been tried but, again, improvements are minimal.

Antioxidants

There is good evidence that active oxygen radicals, present in cigarette smoke, play an important role in damaging the lungs in COPD. They are also released by inflammatory cells such as neutrophils and macrophages. The results of a number of studies have suggested that diets high in fresh fruit and vegetables, which contain many antioxidants, may help to prevent or slow the rate of progress of COPD as well as having favourable effects on various cancers, heart disease and bowel disease. N-Acetyl cysteine is an antioxidant that, in clinical studies, has reduced the number of exacerbations of COPD and, in a two-year uncontrolled study, reduced the rate of decline of FEV_1. More, controlled, studies of the effect of vitamin C and vitamin E in COPD are needed.

Drugs affecting mucus production

N-Acetyl cysteine and similar compounds were developed as mucolytic agents but they are not very effective.

Pulmonary vasodilators

End-stage COPD usually results in pulmonary hypertension secondary to chronic hypoxia. There are no drugs that specifically reduce pulmonary pressure, but the recently developed angiotensin II inhibitor, losartan, reduces pulmonary artery pressure in COPD.

Further reading

BARNES PJ (1998) New therapies for chronic obstructive pulmonary disease. *Thorax* **53**: 137–47.

Organisation and training needs

COPD in primary care is under-diagnosed and under-treated (or over-treated and under-managed). In an average GP list of 2,500 patients there are likely to be 750 smokers (given an average smoking rate of about 30%), of whom 100–150 will have COPD. In areas of social deprivation where smoking rates are higher, the number of COPD patients will be higher. Many of these patients will not be known to their doctor, because they will have mild to moderate disease – so they will be undiagnosed and untreated. On the other hand, many of those whose disease has progressed will be presenting with recurrent chest infections and some will have been misdiagnosed as suffering from asthma – and will be treated for the wrong condition. Those who have severe COPD are likely to be attending hospital and to have been admitted several times with exacerbations of their disease.

Many general practices now offer structured asthma management clinics and it is often the practice nurse who plays a major role. Patients with COPD may have been treated in asthma clinics along asthma management guidelines with ever-increasing doses of expensive asthma therapies. They may have referred themselves, hoping for a new approach to what, too often, is a debilitating disease; or the GP will have referred them, having run out of ideas about what to do for these 'heart sink' patients.

Until recently, there have been no guidelines as to how these patients should be managed, and there has been little training for primary care physicians and nurses. Management tended to be of the 'crisis intervention' variety and there was little understanding of the concepts of proper assessment, diagnosis or long-term management goals for COPD. Patients were frequently given negative advice:

'There is nothing more that I can do for you.'

'I can't give you a new pair of lungs.'

Recently, however, there has been a resurgence of interest in COPD. Guidelines for COPD management have been published by respiratory physician groups around the world. The British version, the BTS Guidelines (published in 1997), have helped to renew interest in COPD in the UK. Recent research has shown that, contrary to previously held beliefs, there are interventions that can improve the quality of life of people with COPD. The proper diagnosis and management of this disease in primary care should result in patients being diagnosed earlier and managed better – and will, hopefully, result in fewer of them being referred for specialist care and repeatedly admitted to hospital. Secondary care is more expensive than primary care and carries a significant risk of infection for people with chronic lung disease.

Patients often prefer not to be admitted to hospital and may find that the GP's surgery is more convenient for them. Structured primary care management may result in:

- fewer emergency general practice consultations,

- the patient and their family having a greater understanding of the disease and improved self-management skills, and

- rational and effective use of medication.

Finding the patients

In order to provide effective management, you must first know who your COPD patients are. It is likely that only those patients with more advanced COPD will be known to you and that many people with moderate disease may have been given an incorrect diagnostic label and are being managed inappropriately. A good starting point, therefore, is to re-examine the practice asthma register, looking particularly at patients over 40 years of age with a current or previous smoking history and who are taking asthma medication. A reassessment of each patient's records and reappraisal of how the diagnosis of asthma was reached may reveal those whose history is more in keeping with a diagnosis of COPD than asthma and those in whom an objective, 'water-tight' diagnosis of asthma is lacking. A synopsis of the features of COPD compared with those of asthma is given in Table 13.1.

The next step is to evaluate the patient's spirometry and to investigate whether there is any reversibility to bronchodilators, as described in Chapter 3.

With patients who do not demonstrate bronchodilator reversibility and are already taking high doses of inhaled steroid but whose history is more suggestive of COPD than asthma, it may be possible to 'wean' them off their steroids, observing the clinical and lung function results.

- Reduce the steroid dose by 25% every three months (as suggested in the BTS *British Guidelines for Asthma Management*).

- Review the patient frequently, observing for rapidly declining lung function or deterioration of symptoms.

- When the patient has been off inhaled steroids for six to eight weeks, conduct a formal oral steroid trial.

Table 13.1 A comparison of the features of COPD and asthma

	COPD	*Asthma*
Onset of symptoms	**Aged 40+ years**	Aged +/– 40 years, 'childhood chestiness' (with or without history of atopic illness)
Smoking history	**15–20+ pack-years**	No or light smoking history
Family history	With or without a history of 'emphysema' 'Chronic bronchitis'	Atopic illness/asthma
Symptoms	**Non-variable** **Shortness of breath on exertion,** cough and sputum with or without wheeze, 'chest tightness'	**Variable** Wheeze, 'chest tightness', cough and sputum in exacerbations
Nocturnal wakening	Rare	**Common**
Morning symptoms	Rapidly relieved by expectoration	Last several hours

The features in **bold** are the particularly relevant ones.

There are no evidence-based guidelines on how to conduct formal steroid trials in patients who are already, and perhaps unnecessarily, taking inhaled steroids. However, the approach outlined above, whilst not giving rapid results, would seem logical. If oral steroids are given to a patient with asthma already optimally controlled on inhaled steroids, any response to the oral steroids is likely to be small and a false-negative result may be obtained. Inhaled steroids may then be stopped when they are in fact needed.

The slow reduction of inhaled steroids, with regular follow-up to ensure that the patient is not deteriorating, may be a safer option. This approach has recently been reinforced by an observational report from the seven-week 'run-in' period of the Isolde trial. Inhaled steroids were withdrawn abruptly before participants were assigned randomly to treatment or placebo in this trial. Over all, 32% of these patients suffered an exacerbation of their COPD during this period.

Considerable savings in the prescribing costs of inhaled steroids can be anticipated by reappraising patients. A survey of nine general practices in 1996 found that 81% of 351 COPD patients were receiving inhaled steroid therapy at a cost of £29,008 over six months. If only the 10–15% of these patients likely to benefit were treated, the cost of inhaled steroid would be reduced to £5,380, a saving of £23,628 in six months.

Reappraisal of the practice asthma register may improve the diagnosis rate in patients with moderate to severe disease and allow more rational prescribing, but it is unlikely to improve the diagnosis rate in patients with mild, largely asymptomatic, disease and those with mild to moderate disease who may be attending with 'chest infections' in the winter. It is an unfortunate fact that, by the time symptoms of COPD become apparent, considerable and irreversible loss of lung function has already occurred. If severe, debilitating, expensive and life-threatening disease is to be prevented, it must be detected early and smoking cessation advice and support given. If awareness of the possibility of COPD is raised with smokers who attend with occasional 'chest infections' and they are screened with spirometry, the detection rate for early COPD is likely to improve.

The role of spirometry in the detection and diagnosis of COPD has already been discussed. However, spirometers are expensive and they must be used properly if the results are not to be meaningless. Incorrectly performed spirometry may result in patients being referred for specialist opinion unnecessarily, or patients needing referral being missed. Training in the correct use and care of equipment and basic interpretation of the results is essential.

A machine that complies with BTS Guidelines for lung function testing and providing the necessary training are likely to cost in excess of £1,000. This may not be practicable for every general practice. Some areas already have open access to spirometry at the local hospital, along similar lines as open access to radiography. This is one of the options suggested by the BTS. The expertise, equipment and facilities for quality control are already available in the hospital, although some extra staffing provision may be needed. Patients, however, may find this less attractive, because it can involve travelling greater distances and thus be less convenient. For a large general practice or a group of smaller practices working co-operatively or a practice with a particular respiratory interest where a machine is likely to be used extensively, the purchase of a spirometer may be a cost-effective option. A third possibility – suggested by the BTS – is the provision of mobile community spirometry services. Which of these options is most the practical must be decided at a local level.

The practice nurse's role

Throughout this book we have emphasised the need for a structured approach to diagnosis and management and the need for patient education, involving both the GP and the practice nurse. Their effectiveness with asthma patients has been widely studied but there is a dearth of research relating to COPD. However, it would seem logical that COPD patients will benefit from a similar approach. The fact that COPD and asthma differ has also been emphasised in this book, to stress how important it is that health professionals caring for patients have a sound understanding of those differences and their implications for treatment.

Providing a structured approach to care in COPD requires doctor or nurse time. In practices already running asthma clinics, extending the scope of the clinic to include COPD management – an 'airways clinic' – is one possible approach. Many COPD patients attend 'asthma clinics', so this may be a practicable option.

Appropriately trained nurses have had – and continue to have – a major impact on asthma management. How involved GPs and nurses are in COPD management should depend on their knowledge, interest and expertise. Whatever their role, they must be trained for it and should have been assessed as competent. The routine care of asthma patients has, in many practices, been almost completely devolved to nurses. However, COPD patients are usually older, often have multiple pathologies and are generally more difficult to manage. They are a group of patients for whom a team approach is essential. Appropriately trained nurses can develop a great deal of expertise in COPD, but may be relatively inexperienced in the management of, for example, ischaemic heart disease, so it is vital that they recognise their limitations (Table 13.2). Easy communication between members of the team and appreciation of each other's expertise and role are needed.

Table 13.2 The role of the practice nurse

Minimum involvement

Maintain a register of known COPD patients

Call COPD patients annually for influenza vaccination

Ensure that COPD patients have received pneumococcal vaccination

Encourage patients to stop smoking, and advise them at each visit

Teach and check inhaler technique

Provide information to patients and their relatives about COPD – e.g. British Lung Foundation

(The patient is managed and followed up by the GP)

Suggested training:

In-house training

Local study evenings in COPD and smoking cessation

+ EXPERIENCE

Medium involvement

As for 'Minimum involvement', plus:

Take a basic respiratory history

Carry out diagnostic procedures – e.g. spirometry and bronchodilator reversibility testing

Update the COPD register

Establish a regular follow-up procedure for COPD patients

Provide basic information and advice on diet and exercise

(The patient is cared for jointly by the GP and the practice nurse)

Training needs:

Training in basic spirometry – know how to care for the equipment and get a technically acceptable result

Basic COPD course – e.g. NARTC COPD Essential Skills Workshop

+ EXPERIENCE

Maximum involvement

As for 'Medium involvement', plus:

Take a full respiratory history

Perform a basic examination of the patient to assess for hyperinflation, central cyanosis and oedema

Be able to recognise abnormal spirometry

Suggest further investigation – chest x-ray, ECG, full blood count, etc.

Assess disability and handicap

Instigate therapeutic trials and evaluate their effectiveness

Assess the need for pulmonary rehabilitation and refer/instigate as necessary

Advise patients on self-management

Liaise with other appropriate health professionals

Provide regular follow-up and support for patients and their families

(The patient is managed and followed up by the nurse, with GP support and advice)

Training needs:

Spirometry interpretation course

An assessed and accredited course in COPD management – e.g. NARTC COPD course

© *The National Asthma and Respiratory Training Centre 1999. Reproduced with permission.*

Protocol and audit

There should be a practice protocol that clearly defines how patients are managed and describes the roles of each member of the primary care team. The protocol should be agreed and followed by all members of the team so that the approach is systematic and logical, and patients receive consistent advice. It should follow the BTS guidelines

Table 13.3 Example of a practice protocol

Case finding and maintenance of disease register

- Update diagnosis opportunistically
- Opportunistic and new patient screening
- Systematic search of patient records (aged 40+, recurrent 'chest infection', smoker)
- Reappraisal of practice asthma register

Diagnostic criteria

- Symptoms
- Lung function – preferably spirometry
- Reversibility to bronchodilators and corticosteroids
- Other investigations – chest x-ray, ECG, full blood count, etc.

Treatment

- Disease severity recorded (post-bronchodilator FEV_1)
- Response to corticosteroids recorded
- Response to therapeutic bronchodilator trials recorded
- Stepwise approach to drug treatment and antibiotics

Referral criteria

- Referral for specialist opinion
- Referral for admission during exacerbation
- Referral for pulmonary rehabilitation (where available)

Follow-up and recall

- Review and recall of patients on practice register
- Follow-up of patients admitted to hospital
- Review of patients on long-term oxygen and nebulisers

Smoking cessation policy

- Record smoking status and 'tag' patient records
- Discuss and encourage the use of nicotine replacement therapy
- Review and recall patients who are 'quitting'

Delegation of care and internal referral policy

- Named GP with overall responsibility
- Role of practice nurse (according to expertise and training)
- Role of support staff

---

for the care of COPD. Suggestions for what should be considered when formulating a practice protocol are given in Table 13.3.

The effectiveness of your practice's COPD management should be audited, so that standards can be maintained and improved, and any deficiencies highlighted and remedied. Unfortunately, there has been little research to determine which outcome measures should be audited, so the suggestions listed in Table 13.4 are largely based on conjecture.

For the health professional the proper management of COPD patients can be immensely rewarding and satisfying. Many patients have been dismissed as 'hopeless cases'. They frequently have low self-esteem and poor expectations. Trevor Clay OBE – former Secretary of the Royal College of Nursing (RCN), tireless campaigner for the British Lung Foundation Breathe Easy groups and a COPD sufferer – summed up the problems many COPD patients face when he addressed the RCN Respiratory Nurses Forum:

'Our [Breathe Easy's] aim is to remove the phrase 'there's nothing more that can be done' from the vocabulary of health professionals. Not only does it have a devastating effect but it is simply not true. What is meant is that there is no magic, no cure, but there is always something that can be done.'

A greater awareness and understanding of COPD should improve the standard of care that COPD patients receive and should ultimately result in a reduction in the burden that this devastating disease causes.

Table 13.4 COPD audit

Audit of process

Percentage of smokers aged 40+ years who have had spirometry performed

Number of COPD patients on the practice register

Percentage of COPD patients who have had an annual review of FEV_1

Audit of outcome

Percentage of COPD patients still smoking

Number of emergency GP consultations

Number of hospital admissions for exacerbations

Improvements in 'disability' scores

Improvements in 'handicap' scores

Further reading

BRITISH THORACIC SOCIETY, ASSOCIATION OF RESPIRATORY TECHNICIANS AND PHYSIOLOGISTS (1994) Guidelines for the measurement of respiratory function. *Respiratory Medicine* **88**: 165–94

BRITISH THORACIC SOCIETY (1997) British guidelines for asthma management. *Thorax* **52** (Suppl 2): S1–34

BRITISH THORACIC SOCIETY (1997) BTS guidelines for the management of chronic obstructive pulmonary disease. *Thorax* **52** (Suppl 5): S1–28

MOUSLEY K, RUDOLPH M, PEARSON M (1996) General practitioner prescribing habits in asthma/COPD. *Thorax* **51** (Suppl 3): 1

Useful addresses

British Lung Foundation
New Garden House
78 Hatton Garden
London EC1N 8LD
Tel: 020 7831 5831

National Asthma and Respiratory Training Centre
The Athenaeum
10 Church Street
Warwick CV34 4AB
Tel: 01926 493313

Glossary

Words shown in *italic* in the definition are also defined in this Glossary

ACE inhibitor angiotensin-converting enzyme inhibitor – a class of drugs used in hypertension and cardiac failure

adaptive aerosol delivery (AAD) an innovative nebuliser system that delivers drug during inhalation only and can be programmed to deliver a precise amount of drug

aerobic exercise exercise to increase the efficiency of the heart and lungs in delivering oxygen to the tissues

air-trapping excess air remaining in the lung at the end of exhalation. This may be due to airway collapse and/or loss of lung elasticity, as in *emphysema*

airway hyper-responsiveness the airways are over-reactive and 'irritable' and more likely to constrict in response to a wide variety of physical and chemical stimuli

alpha-1 antitrypsin (α_1-AT) an *anti-protease* in the blood. Congenital deficiency of alpha-1 antitrypsin is associated with the early presentation (under 40 years of age) of severe *emphysema*

alveolar/capillary interface the surface of the lung where gas exchange occurs

anticholinergic bronchodilator a drug that inhibits the action of acetylcholine on parasympathetic nerve endings in the lungs and dilates airways

antioxidants substances that neutralise oxidants. They occur naturally in foods rich in vitamins C and E, and may help to slow the rate of progression of COPD

antiprotease/elastase enzyme that neutralises protease/elastase (enzymes that destroy lung tissue by digesting *elastin*, one of the proteins that makes up lung parenchyma)

arterial blood gases measurement of the amount of oxygen and carbon dioxide dissolved in the plasma of an arterial blood sample, measured in kilopascals (kPa)

asthma chronic inflammatory condition of the airways, leading to widespread, variable airway obstruction that is reversible spontaneously or with treatment. Long-standing asthma may become unresponsive to treatment

atopy hereditary predisposition to develop allergic *asthma*, rhinitis and eczema. It is associated with high levels of the antibody IgE

beta-agonist bronchodilator a drug that stimulates the beta-adrenergic receptors in the lungs, resulting in bronchodilation

Blue Badge (formerly **Orange Badge**) **scheme** a scheme for disabled persons, allowing them to park in restricted areas

'blue bloater' a somewhat outmoded term used to describe a cyanosed COPD patient who is oedematous and at risk of *cor pulmonale*

Borg scale a measure of breathlessness by which the patient quantifies the amount of breathlessness that an activity produces

breath-assisted nebuliser a jet nebuliser that boosts output during inhalation and minimises drug wastage during exhalation

Breathe Easy the name of patient support groups facilitated by the British Lung Foundation

bronchiectasis irreversible dilation of the bronchi due to bronchial wall damage, causing chronic cough and mucopurulent sputum

broncho-alveolar lavage a technique used to wash samples of cells from small airways and alveoli. It is performed during bronchoscopy

bronchomotor tone the amount of bronchial muscle contraction (tone) normally present in the airways. This is often increased in COPD patients

bullous emphysema large cyst-like spaces in the lung that compress normal lung tissue. It may be amenable to surgery

chronic bronchitis sputum production that occurs on most days for at least three months in at least two consecutive years (Medical Research Council definition)

chronic obstructive pulmonary disease (COPD) a slowly progressive disorder characterised by airflow obstruction, which does not change markedly over several months (British Thoracic Society definition)

collagen a connective tissue. Deposition of collagen in the basement membrane of small airways contributes to irreversible airflow obstruction

cor pulmonale pulmonary hypertension and right ventricular hypertrophy (and eventual failure) occurring as a result of chronic lung disease. It causes peripheral oedema, raised jugular venous pressure and liver enlargement

corticosteroid reversibility a test done to determine which COPD patients have significant response (an increase in FEV_1 greater than 200ml and 15% of baseline) to steroids and who merit long-term inhaled steroids. Large improvements are indicative of *asthma* rather than COPD. Prednisolone 30mg is given in the morning for 2 weeks. Alternatively 1,000μg per day of beclomethasone (or equivalent) is given for 6 weeks

corticosteroids/steroids hormones produced by the adrenal glands. Synthetic forms are used in COPD for their anti-inflammatory activity, although their long-term use is controversial

cyanosis blueness of the skin due to *hypoxia*. It is a somewhat subjective finding but when oxygen saturation falls below 85–90% cyanosis generally becomes apparent

cyclic adenosine monophosphate (cyclic AMP) a substance found in cells that has a crucial role in bronchodilation and reduction of inflammation

cytokines glycoprotein molecules that regulate cell-to-cell communication of the inflammatory response

dynamic airway collapse the tendency of unsupported airways to collapse during forced exhalation

elastase enzyme that digests *elastin*

elastin protein that makes up lung tissue. Its elastic properties contribute to the lung's elastic recoil and helps expel air from the lungs during exhalation

emphysema abnormal permanent enlargement of the air spaces distal to the terminal bronchiole (alveoli) accompanied by destruction of their walls

eosinophil white blood cell. It is characteristically found in the airways of people with *asthma* and is implicated in long-term inflammation and epithelial damage

FEV₁ see *forced expired volume*

fibrosing alveolitis a condition resulting in widespread *fibrosis* of the alveoli. It causes progressive breathlessness and a restrictive spirometry pattern

fibrosis scarring and thickening of an organ or tissue by replacement of the original tissue with collagenous fibrous tissue

flow/volume trace a graph produced by a spirometer in which flow rate (in litres per second) is on the vertical axis and volume (in litres) on the horizontal axis

forced expired volume (FEV₁) the amount of air that can be exhaled in the first second of a forced blow from maximum inhalation

forced vital capacity (FVC) the total volume of air that can be exhaled from a maximal inhalation to maximal exhalation

gas transfer test (TLco) a test performed in lung function laboratories that determines the ability of the lungs to take up a small amount of carbon monoxide. It is a measure of how efficiently the *alveolar/capillary interface* is working

'guy-rope effect' the support given to small airways by the elastic walls of the alveoli in the lung parenchyma

health status/quality of life a measure of the impact of a disease on a patient's daily life, and social and emotional well-being

Hoover's sign in-drawing of the lower intercostal margins on inhalation

hypercapnia high levels of carbon dioxide in the blood. Levels over 6kPa are generally considered to be abnormal

hypoxia low levels of oxygen in the blood. Levels below 10kPa are generally considered to be abnormal

hypoxic challenge a method of assessing the response of a patient to the reduced oxygen levels they will encounter during air travel

hypoxic respiratory drive a stimulus to breathe that is driven by low levels of oxygen. When patients with this abnormal drive are given high levels of oxygen the stimulus to breathe will be suppressed, resulting in worsening respiratory failure or respiratory arrest

immunoglobulin E (IgE) an antibody. Raised levels of IgE are associated with *atopy* and allergy

inhaled corticosteroids/steroids *corticosteroids* available as beclomethasone, budesonide or fluticasone in a variety of inhaler devices

jet nebulisers the most commonly used nebuliser. Atomising the drug solution in the airflow from a compressor or piped gas supply produces the aerosol

leukotriene antagonists a new class of drugs for *asthma* that either block the formation of leukotrienes or block the leukotriene receptors in the lungs

long-term oxygen therapy (LTOT) oxygen given for 15 hours or more a day. It improves life expectancy and may improve health status in chronically hypoxic COPD patients

losartan a recently developed angiotensin II inhibitor that reduces pulmonary artery pressure in COPD

lung volume reduction surgery a new technique developed in the USA to remove 20–30% of the most emphysematous parts of the lung and improve breathlessness

lymphocytes white blood cells involved in the body's immune system

macrophages white blood cells that are involved in phagocytosis and secretion of cytokines that attract and activate neutrophils and other inflammatory cells

mast cells white blood cells that release histamine and other inflammatory mediators. *Immunoglobulin E* is attached to their surfaces

nicotine replacement therapy (NRT) a method of reducing craving and withdrawal symptoms in people attempting to stop smoking. It is available as chewing gum, transdermal patches, inhalator, nasal spray and sublingual tablets. It can double success rates

obliterative bronchiolitis widespread fibrotic, inflammatory condition of the small airways. A late and serious complication of lung transplantation, it is frequently fatal in 6–12 months

obstructive sleep apnoea (OSA) upper airway obstruction occurring during sleep. It may result in repeated and significant episodes of hypoxia and severe sleep deprivation. Can cause *cor pulmonale* and may coexist with COPD. Commonly presents with daytime somnolence and a history of severe snoring

occupational asthma variable airway obstruction resulting from exposure to a sensitising agent inhaled at work. Continued exposure to the causative agent may result in severe, persistent *asthma* with irreversibility

osteoporosis demineralisation and atrophy of bone, associated with an increased risk of fracture. It is most commonly seen in post-menopausal women but is also associated with long-term use of oral *corticosteroids*

oxidants see *oxygen radicals/oxidants*

oxygen concentrator electrically powered molecular 'sieve' that removes nitrogen and carbon dioxide and delivers almost pure oxygen to the patient. It is a cost-effective method of delivering long-term oxygen

oxygen cost diagram a measure of disability in which a patient marks a 10cm line against an activity that induces breathlessness. The disability score is the distance along the line

oxygen radicals/oxidants highly active molecules – found in tobacco smoke and released by inflammatory cells – that can damage lung tissue

oxygen saturation the percentage of haemoglobin saturated with oxygen. It is measured with a pulse oximeter. Normal oxygen saturation is over 95%. Cyanosis is apparent with a saturation of between 85% and 90%

peak expiratory flow (PEF) the maximal flow rate that can be maintained over the first 10 milliseconds of a forced blow

phosphodiesterase inhibitors a group of drugs, including *theophyllines*, that increase *cyclic AMP* levels and may reduce inflammation and cause bronchodilation

photochemical pollutants gases such as ozone, produced by the action of sunlight on vehicle exhaust gases

'pink puffer' a somewhat outmoded term to describe a COPD patient who is very breathless but has normal arterial blood gases and is not at risk of the early development of *cor pulmonale*

pneumococcal vaccination recommended for COPD patients by the Department of Health although controlled studies of its effectiveness are lacking

pneumotachograph a device for measuring flow rates. Some electronic spirometers use these to assess flow rates and calculate lung volumes from the flow rates

polycythaemia an abnormal increase in the number of red blood cells. In COPD this can occur as a result of chronic *hypoxia*

pulmonary oedema extravasated fluid in the lung tissue. Commonly caused by left ventricular failure

pulmonary rehabilitation a programme of exercises and education aimed at reducing disability and handicap in chronic respiratory disease.

pulse oximetry a non-invasive method of assessing the amount of haemoglobin that is saturated with oxygen (*oxygen saturation*)

quality of life see *health status*

respiratory drive the stimulus to breathe. The main respiratory centre is in the medulla of the brain

respiratory failure failure to maintain oxygenation. It is usually taken to mean failure to maintain oxygenation above 8kPa

respiratory muscle training breathing exercises aimed at improving respiratory muscle strength and endurance. Its effectiveness in COPD is debatable

restrictive lung disease a disease that causes reduction in lung volumes (FVC and FEV_1) without reduction in flow rates through the airways (FEV_1/FVC ratio normal or high)

sarcoid an inflammatory disease of unknown cause affecting many parts of the body. Chronic sarcoidosis affecting the lungs causes diffuse fibrosis, reduction of lung volumes and, sometimes, airflow obstruction with air-trapping

shuttle walking test a method of assessing walking distance. The patient performs a paced walk between two points 10 metres apart (a shuttle) at an incrementally increasing pace, dictated by 'beeps' on a tape recording, until they are unable to maintain the pace

'silent area' a term used to describe the generation of airways 2–5mm in diameter. Considerable damage can occur in this area without causing symptoms

simple bronchitis chronic mucus production that is not associated with airflow obstruction

small airways disease pathological changes affecting airways 2–5mm in diameter, including occlusion of the airway with mucus, goblet cell hyperplasia, inflammatory changes in the airway wall, fibrosis and smooth muscle hypertrophy

smoking 'pack-years' a method of quantifying cigarette exposure:

$$\frac{\text{Number smoked per day}}{20} \times \text{Number of years smoked}$$

steroids see *corticosteroids*

theophyllines methylxanthine bronchodilator drug with a modest bronchodilator effect in COPD

total lung capacity (TLC) the volume of air in the lungs after maximum inhalation. It comprises the vital capacity and the residual volume

ultrasonic nebulisers nebulisers in which the aerosol is generated by agitating the nebuliser solution with ultrasonic vibrations produced by a piezo crystal

ventilation/perfusion mismatch a situation in which areas of the lung have a blood supply and no air and vice versa. It results in inefficient gas exchange

Venturi mask an oxygen mask that supplies a fixed percentage of oxygen

volume/time trace a graph produced by a spirometer whereby volume is plotted on the vertical axis and time on the horizontal axis

Useful addresses

Breathe Easy
British Lung Foundation
78 Hatton Garden
London EC1N 8LD
Tel: 020 7831 5831
*Self-help groups for social
contact, support and
encouragement*

British Lung Foundation
New Garden House
78 Hatton Garden
London EC1N 8LD
Tel: 020 7831 5831
*For leaflets containing
information about suitable
gentle exercises and breathing
control*

**Chest, Heart and Stroke
Association (Northern Ireland)**
21 Dublin Road
Belfast BT2 7HB
Tel: 028 90 320184
For information and advice

**Chest, Heart and Stroke
Association (Scotland)**
65 North Castle Street
Edinburgh EH2 3LT
Tel: 0131 225 6963
For information and advice

Health Education Authority
Trevelyan House
30 Great Peter Street
London SW1P 2HW
Tel: 020 7222 5300
*For details of a wide range of
leaflets and books promoting
good health*

**National Asthma and
Respiratory Training Centre**
The Athenaeum
10 Church Street
Warwick CV34 4AB
Tel: 01926 493313
*Courses on respiratory care for
all health professionals.
Publications:* Simply COPD,
Simply Stop Smoking

**Quitline (Smokeline in
Scotland)**
England: 0800 00 22 00
Northern Ireland:
028 90 663 281
Scotland: 0800 84 84 84
Wales: 0345 697 500
*For help with trying to stop
smoking*

Addresses for breathlessness questionnaires

Chronic Respiratory Disease Index Questionnaire
Gordon Guyatt
Department of Clinical
Epidemiology and Biostatistics
McMaster University Medical
Centre
1200 Main Street West
Hamilton, Ontario, CANADA
L8N 3Z5

St George's Respiratory Questionnaire
Professor Paul Jones
Division of Physiological
Medicine
St George's Hospital Medical
School
Cranmer Terrace
London SW17 0RE

Breathing Problems Questionnaire
Professor Michael Hyland
Department of Psychology
University of Plymouth
Plymouth
Devon PL4 8AA

Manufacturers

3M Health Care Ltd
3M House
Morley Street
Loughborough
Leicestershire LE11 1EP
Tel: 01509 611611

Allen & Hanburys Ltd
Stockley Park West
Uxbridge
Middlesex UB11 1BT
Tel: 020 8990 9888

Astra Zeneca
Home Park Estate
Kings Langley
Herts WD4 8DH
Tel: 01923 266191

Baker Norton
Albert Basin
Armada Way
Royal Docks
London E16 2QJ
Tel: 08705 020304

Boehringer Ingelheim Ltd
Ellesfield Avenue
Southern Industrial Estate
Bracknell
Berkshire RG12 8YS
Tel: 01344 424600

Clement Clarke
International Ltd
Unit A
Cartel Business Estate
Edinburgh Way
Harlow
Essex CM20 2TT
Tel: 01279 414969

Ferraris Medical Ltd
Aden Road
Enfield
Middlesex EN3 7SE
Tel: 020 8805 9055

Glaxo Wellcome
Stockley Park West
Uxbridge
Middlesex UB11 1BT
Tel: 020 8990 9888

Medic-Aid Ltd
Heath Place
Bognor Regis
West Sussex PO22 9SL
Tel: 01243 840888

Micro Medical
PO Box 6
Rochester
Kent ME1 2AZ
Tel: 01634 360044

Napp Pharmaceuticals
Cambridge Science Park
Milton Road
Cambridge CB4 0GW
Tel: 01223 424444

Rhone-Poulenc Rorer Ltd
RPR House
50 Kings Hill Avenue
Kings Hill
West Malling
Kent ME19 4AH
Tel: 01732 584000

Vitalograph Ltd
Maids Moreton House
Maids Moreton
Buckingham MK18 1SW
Tel: 01280 827110

Index

Have you found *COPD in Primary Care* helpful? Then you may be interested in these other books from Class Health.

Asthma at your fingertips £14.99
Dr Mark Levy, Professor Sean Hilton and Greta Barnes MBE

This exceptional book, written by three leading experts, is the one you will want to recommend to your patients. Written in an user-friendly question and answer style, it shows them how to keep their asthma under control, and how to lead a full, happy and healthy life with asthma.

Asthma: ask the experts £24.99
Edited by Greta Barnes, NARTC

Published to mark the 10th anniversary of the National Asthma and Respiratory Training Centre, this book brings together the knowledge and experience of over 100 experts on asthma. Included among the book's contributors are eminent hospital physicians, general practitioners, specialist asthma nurses, pharmacologists and psychologists. A highly readable account of every aspect of asthma management.

Allergies at your fingertips £14.99
Dr Joanne Clough

At last – sensible practical advice on allergies from an experienced medical expert. Dr Clough answers over 300 real questions from people with allergies and their families, giving you advice you can trust.

'An excellent book which deserves to be on the bookshelf of every family.' – *Dr Csaba Rusznak, Medical and Scientific Director, British Allergy Foundation*

**Eczema and your child:
a parent's guide** £11.99
Dr Tim Mitchell, Dr David Paige and Karen Spowart
Three acknowledged experts in the field answer the questions that concern parents whose children have eczema.

This practical and positive handbook is one you can recommend to your patients with confidence.

Vital Diabetes £14.99
Dr Charles Fox and Mary MacKinnon

Your essential reference for diabetes management in primary care. You know just how hard it is to remember everything you need to manage diabetes in general practice. Things change fast in diabetes and it is hard to keep all the new information at your fingertips. This book gives you all the latest up-to-date and essential information – in just 96 pages!

**Providing diabetes care
in general practice** £21.95
Mary MacKinnon

The new third edition of the 'bible' for primary care diabetes. This book gives you all the back-up and information you need to run a high-quality, effective diabetes service within your practice.

'The complete guide for the primary care team.' – *Dr Michael Hall, Chairman of the BDA.*

Diabetes in the real world £21.95
Dr Charles Fox and Dr Tony Pickering

Confronts the issues and problems of diabetes care in general practice, from the perspective of the GP at the coal face. This DIY manual gives you confidence in dealing with all the diabetic issues in your practice. It deals with the questions that occur daily in the real world of general practice – rather than the artificially ordered environment of the textbook.

PRIORITY ORDER FORM

Please cut out or photocopy this form and send it to:
Class Publishing (Priority Service)
FREEPOST (PAM 6219) (*no stamp required if posted in the UK*),
Plymouth PL6 7ZZ
URGENT – please send me the following books: (*enter quantity below*)

No. of copies		Price including p&p
☐	*COPD in Primary Care* (1 872362 95 8)	£27.99
☐	*Asthma at your fingertips* (1 872362 67 2)	£17.99
☐	*Asthma: ask the experts* (1 872362 68 0)	£27.99
☐	*Allergies at your fingertips* (1 872362 52 4)	£17.99
☐	*Eczema and your child: a parent's guide* (1 872362 86 9)	£14.99
☐	*Vital Diabetes* (1 872362 78 8)	£17.99
☐	*Providing diabetes care in general practice* (1 872362 74 5)	£24.95
☐	*Diabetes in the real world* (1 872362 53 2)	£22.95
☐	Please send me further details about these books (✓)	

Please note all prices include UK postage and handling costs.

For express service, use our Hotlines:
☎ 01752 202 301   Fax: 01752 202 333

EASY WAYS TO PAY

1. I enclose a cheque made payable to Class Publishing for _____

2. Please charge my   Access ☐   Visa ☐   Switch ☐   Amex ☐

Card no. _____   Expiry date _____

Name _____   Occupation _____

Delivery address _____

_____

Daytime telephone (*in case of query*) _____

Send to: **Class Publishing (Priority Service), FREEPOST (PAM 6219),**
Plymouth PL6 7ZZ
Or use one of the Hotlines listed above

Publisher's no quibble guarantee: your money back in full
if you are not entirely satisfied within 30 days of receipt.